INDEPENDENT LIVING & DISABILITY POLICY IN THE NETHERLANDS: THREE MODELS OF RESIDENTIAL CARE & INDEPENDENT LIVING

by
Gerben DeJong, Ph.D.

**Senior Research Associate
& Associate Professor
Department of Rehabilitation Medicine
Tufts University School of Medicine
Tufts-New England Medical Center
Boston, Massachusetts
U.S.A.**

**Senior Fulbright Scholar
Sociale Verzekeringsraad
Zoetermeer
The Netherlands**

International Exchange of Experts and Information in Rehabilitation
World Rehabilitation Fund, Inc.
400 East 34th Street
New York, New York 10016

This investigation was supported in part by (1) the World Rehabilitation Fund under a grant (no. G00 8103982) from the National Institute of Handicapped Research, U.S. Department of Education, Washington, DC 20201; and (2) the Fulbright Program administered by the Council for the International Exchange of Scholars, Washington, DC 20036, and the Netherlands America Commission for Educational Exchange, 1017 DG Amsterdam. under a grant from the U.S. International Communication Agency, Washington, DC.

ISBN #939986-40-X

ACKNOWLEDGEMENTS

The research for this monograph was initiated with a grant from the World Rehabilitation Fund of New York which enabled me to carry out a fellowship visit to the Netherlands in late 1982. In 1984, I was fortunate to return under the auspices of the Fulbright program for a more extended stay that allowed me to expand the original focus of the research and prepare this monograph.

This monograph would not have been possible without the support of several key persons and their respective organizations. First, I should mention Ms. Diane Woods, Project Director for the World Rehabilitation Fund's International Exchange of Experts and Information in Rehabilitation program in New York. Without her support and patience this publication never would have materialized. Second, I would like to acknowledge Ms. Johanna Wind, Executive Director of the Fulbright Commision in Amsterdam. She and her staff did much to facilitate my stay in the Netherlands and to make it the educational experience that it was. Third, I would like to thank drs. Pieter Stroink, Chief of the Research & Behavioral Science Division within the Medical Affairs Section of Holland's Social Security Council in Zoetermeer. Drs. Stroink graciously served as my host for the duration of the study and made the resources of his staff available to me. Members of his staff proved to be an invaluable resource. In this regard, I should mention drs. Michael Herweyer whose knowledge of the Dutch social insurance system and public policy process proved indispensable.

A number of persons consented to review the manuscript for accuracy. They include drs. Michael Herweyer introduced above; Mr. Jan van Leer formerly of the National Organization for Disability Policy; Ms. J.S. Frijda of the Central Council for Home Help Services; Mr. G. Heykamp of the Fokus Foundation; Mr. J. Hendricks, a self-employed psychologist in Utrecht; and Dr. Adolf Ratska of the Institute of Technology, School of Architecture and Planning, Stockholm, Sweden.

Altogether, more than 50 interviews were conducted in the course of the study. Many individuals gave generously of their time. Because they are too numerous to mention here, they are listed in the appendix.

Not to be overlooked in this array of acknowledgments are my colleagues in the Department of Rehabilitation Medicine at Tufts who kept the home fires burning. I would also like to acknowledge my department chairman, Dr. B. Gans for his backing.

The shortcomings of this monograph are entirely my own. In no way are they to reflect on the World Rehabilitation Fund, the Fulbright Commission, the Dutch Social Security Council, or the reviewers mentioned above.

Gerben DeJong, Ph.D.
Zoetermeer/Leiden
The Netherlands
Spring 1984

TABLE OF CONTENTS

TABLE OF CONTENTS (Continued)

NOTE TO THE READER

This monograph was written primarily for an American audience. However, working in 2 languages always presents a problem when a term or concept does not translate well from the first language (in this case, Dutch) into the second language (in this case, English). To cope with this problem, I have used a convention that has become quite common in cross-national literature, i.e., using a translation that communicates best with the intended audience, followed by an italicized rendition of the original term or concept in parentheses. This convention was also used to minimize any potential misunderstandings with the monograph's Dutch readership.

Although I have tried to avoid using acronyms and abbreviations, there are many multisyllabic Dutch terms that are either long or simply awkward to translate. In such cases, I have resorted to using an acronym or an abbreviation. However, so as not to use yet another set of acronyms or abbreviations, I have opted for using the Dutch acronym—but only after or when the Dutch term and its best available translation have been used. This procedure was decided upon after considering (1) the potential for confusion and (2) the needs of both American and Dutch audiences. The use of Dutch acronyms is used mainly in discussions involving Dutch disability laws and organizations. A list of all abbreviations is provided on the next page.

Another problem arises with the terms "disabled" and "handicapped" which are used differently in the Netherlands and the United States. In the Netherlands the term "disabled" (*ongeschikheid*) is usually used in discussions relating to work disability and disability compensation. The term "handicapped" (*gehandicap*) is usually used in discussions involving severe disability. However, in the United States, the term "disabled" has become the more common term and the term preferred by persons with disabilities. It is also the term used here.

After completing a study of this scope, one cannot help but have opinions about the Dutch disability and independent living systems. Throughout the document, except in Sections IV and V, I have tried, but have not always succeeded, to avoid making opinions or recommendations about the Dutch system, especially when one intent of the monograph is to consider the implications of the Dutch system for the United States. However, when comparative analysis is called for, value judgments are nearly impossible to avoid. This is especially the case in Sections IV and V.

Sometimes values and opinions are simply implicit in the whole manner of one's analysis. Therefore I should make clear that my understanding of disability issues arises from several disciplinary perspectives—economics, political science, medical rehabilitation, and policy research—within an American context. But more importantly, my understanding of disability issues has been shaped in a significant way by the perspective and values of the American independent living movement. Nonetheless, I have tried to remain cognizant of those features of the movement that are distinctively American in origin and thus not always applicable to another country with a somewhat different value system.

The Author

ABBREVIATIONS

AAW   Algemene Arbeidsongeschikheids Wet
(General Work Disability Law)

ABP   Algemeen Burgerlijke Pensioenfond
(General Public Sector Pension Act)

ABW   Algemene Bijstandwet
(General Assistance Act)

ADL   Algemene dagelijke levensverrichtingen
(General activities of daily living)

ANIB   algemene Nederlandse Invalid Bond
(general Dutch Disability Alliance)

ARP   Anti-Revolutionary Party

AWBZ   Algemene Wet Bijzondere Ziektekosten
(General Exceptional Medical Expenses Act)

CRM   Ministerie van Cultuur, Recreatie, & Maatschapelijk Werk
(Ministry of Culture, Recreation, & Social Work)

GAK   Gemeenscappelijk Administratie Kantoor
(Joint Administrative Office)

GMD   Gemeenschappelijke Medische Dienst
(Joint Medical Service)

GON   Gehandicapten Organatie van Nederland
(Organization of the Disabled in the Netherlands)

GR   Nederlandse Gehandicaptenraad
(Dutch Handicapped Council)

IL   independent living

KVP   Katholieke Volks Partij
(Catholic Peoples Party)

NOG   Nationaal Orgaan Gehandicaptenbeleid
(National Organization for Disability Policy)

NOZ   National Organization for the Care of the Mentally Retarded

NVR   Nederlandse Verenigingen voor Revalidatie
(Dutch Rehabilitation Association)

PI   particulier initiatief
(private initiative)

PvdA   Partij van de Arbeid
(Labor Party)

SVR   Sociale Verzekeringsraad
        (Social Insurance Council)

SZ   Ministerie van Sociale Zaken
        (Ministry of Social Affairs)

SZW   Ministerie van Sociale Zaken & Wekgelegenheid
        (Ministry of Social Affairs & Employment)

VROM   Ministerie van Volkshuisvesting, Ruimtelijke Ordening, & Milieuhy-
        giene
        (Ministry of Housing, Land Use Planning, & Environment)

VVD   Volkspartij voor Vrijheid en Democratie
        (Liberal Party)

WAO   Wet op de Arbeidsongeschikheidsverzekering
        (Work Disability Insurance Act)

WVC   Ministerie van Welzijn, Volksgezondheid, & Cultuur
        (Ministry of Welfare, Public Health, & Culture)

ZFR   Ziekenfondsraad
        (Health Insurance Council)

ZFW   Ziekenfondswet
        (Sickness Fund Law)

ZW   Ziektewet
        (Sickness Benefit Act)

I INTRODUCTION

The United States and the Netherlands have embarked on somewhat different courses in seeking to meet the independent living aspirations of people with physical disabilities. The American independent living (IL) movement has focused on the IL Center as the principal coordinating vehicle by which persons with disabilities can through self-advocacy and self-help organize the various housing, transportation, and attendant care services they need to live independently in the community. The Dutch system by contrast has focused on a 3-part network of quasi-residential and IL programs, often under private sponsorship, but more firmly linked to the nation's various entitlement programs.

There is no such thing as an IL center in the Netherlands. This is not to suggest that the disability rights movement in the Netherlands is at an arrested state of development. Rather it reflects the fact that the IL needs of disabled Dutch citizens have been more readily embraced by Holland's mainstream entitlement programs. In the United States, the IL needs of disabled persons have been addressed at the periphery of American disability-related entitlement programs. IL centers came to be in the United States, in part, as the result of the failure of mainline programs to address the needs of persons with physical disabilities. In many respects, IL centers were spawned to compensate for shortcomings in the larger American health and human service system.

Scope and Purpose of the Monograph

This monograph critically examines how Holland's 3-part system of residential care and independent living is wedded to the country's mainline health and social welfare systems giving due consideration to the larger economic, social, and political context in which Holland's various programs have emerged. By anchoring residential and IL programs within the framework of its various entitlement programs, the Netherlands has helped to provide a relatively secure funding base for its residential and IL system. However, in doing so, providers and consumers are also presented with a variety of economic and programmatic incentives that can sometimes work at cross purposes. My purpose is to examine the factors and incentives that have given rise to the present residential and IL system, and how some of its best features can be applied to the United States.

In keeping with the scope and purpose of this monograph, Section II explores the larger economic, social, and political context in which Dutch disability and IL policy has been shaped giving particular attention to the influence of Holland's highly ''confessionalized'' past. Section III outlines the scope of Holland's social insurance system as it relates to the needs of persons with severe physical disabilities. Section IV compares and contrasts each of the 3 main models of residential care and independent living. In this section special attention is given to the manner in which attendant care—or what the Dutch call ''ADL assistance''—is provided in different settings. Section V evaluates Holland's 3 models as a system that is undergoing varying degrees of stress in response to funding cutbacks and in response to a heightened sense of competition between the various models. This section speculates on the near term future of the 3 models and considers their implications for the United States.

I do not want to suggest that the learning process should be a one-way street, from the Netherlands to the United States. Curiously enough, as we shall see, the Dutch can be locked into their own models and ways of doing things that limit options for persons with disabilities. Nonetheless, the Dutch have made a commitment to making sure that disabled persons share in Holland's overall postwar prosperity—not through ''trickle-down'' economics, but through deliberate resource allocation decisions. However, as we shall also see, that commitment is being put to a severe test as a result of the 1980's recession which has pushed unemloyment rates in the Netherlands to as high as 15%.

Introducing Holland's 3-part System

At the risk of oversimplifying matters, Holland's residential and IL system can be viewed as a continuum consisting of 3 main alternatives or models ranked from least independent to most independent (see Figure 1-1):
    (1) The residential center model (*woonvormen*)
        A. Large residential centers (*grote woonvormen*)
        B. Small residential centers (*kleine woonvormen*)
    (2) The clustered housing model (*Fokus projecten*)
    (3) The independent housing model (*op zich zelf wonen*)
Although each model has its own origins and special sponsorship, collectively they may be viewed as a system of living alternatives that is highly interac-

tive: policies initiated in one component of the system are likely to affect other components of the system. A brief description of each follows:

The residential center model is comprised of both large and small residential centers that differ mainly in scale than in program or governance:

Figure 1-1
Residential & IL Alternatives
in the Netherlands

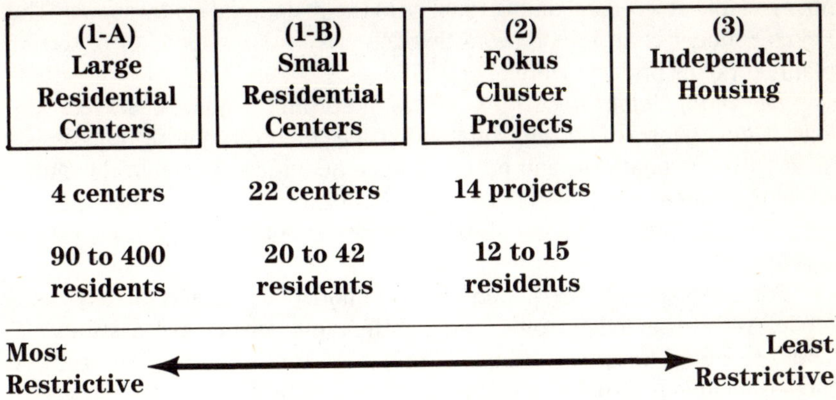

Large residential centers accommodate between 90 and 450 residents. Each resident has his/her own dwelling with a separate mailing address. Meals can be eaten communally or in one's own residence. Attendant care is obtained from a nonuniformed central staff. Each resident has considerable autonomy, however, most day-to-day affairs of the center are directed by the staff. There is usually a residents' council whose decision making powers are more akin to that of a college student council in the United States. Nationally and internationally, the best-known and largest center of this kind is Het Dorp located near Arnhem. There are four large centers of this kind in the Netherlands.

Small residential centers are very much like the larger residential centers except that they accommodate 20 to 42 residents each. Although individual dwellings are usually larger than in the large residential centers, the range of services and the governance of the smaller centers are not much different than their larger counterparts. There are 22 small residential centers of this type. Most of these centers are paired up with a "day activity center" usually located a few kilometers away. Each resident is expected to participate in such a center or to be involved in the community by participating in gainful work or in volunteer activities.

The clustered housing model, hereafter referred to as Fokus projects, is the latest rage in the Netherlands. Each Fokus project accommodates 12 to 15 residents who rent their own apartments in scattered locations throughout a large newly built housing development. From the outside, Fokus dwellings are indistinguishable from other apartments in the housing development. Attendant care can be acquired from a central station of "ADL assistants." If needed, assistance with housekeeping activities must be acquired from non-Fokus sources. Each resident is responsible for his/her own meals; meals are not available at a central dining room as in the residential center model. The Fokus concept is an import from Sweden. As of early 1984, 14 of the 35 planned Fokus projects were operational.

The independent housing model is, according to some observers, the least common form of housing for working age persons requiring daily assistance with personal care and other in-home activities. Although the Dutch social insurance system will make a number of services available to individuals living in their own home, attendant care is not routinely among these services.

For purposes of this paper, the common denominator across these models is the disabled person's need for attendant care or "ADL assistance." Thus, the most common disabling conditions represented in these three models include post-polio, spinal cord injury, cerebral palsy, multiple sclerosis, spina bifida, and other neuromuscular conditions.[1]

Additional Considerations

Some American readers will object to including the residential center model as part of an overall discussion on independent living in the Netherlands. Some would also extend that objection to Fokus. As an observer of the American IL movement, I agree that the objection has considerable foundation; the residential center model is, first and foremost, an institutional model, not an IL model. However, 3 observations are in order.

First, the residential center model is important from an historical and evolutionary perspective. Traces of earlier approaches can be found in the present array of services to persons with disabilities. The Dutch system has undergone considerable change over the last 20 years and continues to change in the present. Yet, the residential model looms large and simply cannot be ignored as an important part of the spectrum of services currently available to Holland's disabled citizens.

---

1. *These have also been the major disability groups represented in the IL movement in the United States. However, one tends to observe a greater variety of disabling conditions and a greater range of age groups among persons participating in Holland's 3-part residential and IL system.*

14

Second, even some of Holland's largest residential centers provide for substantial personal autonomy and respect for individual personhood that cannot be found in comparably sized programs in the United States. They are not like American nursing homes. Residential centers do have objectionable trappings and these will be noted elsewhere in this monograph.

Third, the Dutch are accustomed to living at close quarters. As such the Dutch have a stronger tradition of planning and developing group-based solutions to vexing social and economic problems in face of scarce land and high density living. For example, Fokus projects are an intricate part of a much larger land use planning effort in each of the communities in which projects have sprung up. Likewise, a casual American could easily object to how some dwellings in a residential center are spaced, failing to take note of the fact that row housing is fairly typical of most Dutch cities and villages.

It's been said by some foreign observers that many elements of the American IL movement strongly reflect the American sense of individualism, with its model of the totally independent all-sufficient person. Although only few of us ever attain that level of independence, many of our views, of how persons with disabilities should live, are driven by this model. What we fail to realize is that in another culture, the American model of independence may not be the way to self-direction and personal autonomy so essential to the definition of personhood.

I do not wish to offer an apology for what might be considered shortcomings in the Dutch system of alternatives for persons with disabilities. However, one does need to take cognizance of the cultural values and assumptions he/she takes to a subject such as independent living in another country. Complacent smugness denies a person the opportunity to learn from the observations that may otherwise have been casually written off as irrelevant.

II THE LARGER DEMOGRAPHIC, ECONOMIC, SOCIAL & POLITICAL CONTEXT

Much of the Dutch residential care and IL system cannot be understood apart from the larger demographic, economic, social, and political context in which the system has arisen. Nor can the implications of the system for other countries such as the United States be fully ascertained without this prior knowledge. This section of the monograph trys to provide the reader with just enough background information to gain a better grasp of the various forces within Dutch society that have helped to shape the Dutch disability and IL policy as it is known today.

Some may find this discussion to be a digression. However, the important role of various demographic, economic, social, and political forces cannot be overstated and are essential to the discussion that follows.

THE DEMOGRAPHIC CONTEXT

The Netherlands is a country of 14.3 million people crammed into about 13,000 square miles making it one of the most densely populated countries in the world, second only to Bangledesh. Population density and land scarcity have done much to shape both land use planning and social policy. For example, housing for disabled persons is very much linked to urban land use planning and development.

Demographic Diversity

One of the most often heard remarks made by Americans is that the Netherlands is a homogeneous country with little ethnic, racial, or religious diversity. The remark is often volunteered as a way of suggesting that little within the Netherlands could be applied to a country as diverse and heterogeneous as the United States. It is also volunteered as a way of suggesting that American social and economic problems are more intractable because of its diversity and therefore less should be expected of American public policy in addressing the needs of more vulnerable groups such as persons with disabilities.

A few statistics should help to dispell such thinking. For example, 40% of the children in the Rotterdam school system are foreign born or of foreign parentage and must learn Dutch as a second language. Because of labor shortages in the postwar economy, the Netherlands "imported" a large number of foreign workers from Morroco, Tunisia, Spain, Italy, Turkey, and other countries. Many of these workers and their respective families have elected to remain in the Netherlands. Moreover, the Netherlands has had to cope with the legacy of its former colonial empire by absorbing numerous individuals from places such as Indonesia, the Netherlands Antilles, and Surinam. In 1975, when Surinam declared its independence, some 60,000 persons (mainly Creoles and Hindustanis) migrated to the Netherlands. Today there are about 180,000 Surinamers living in the Netherlands (Muus, et al., 1983; Centraal Bureau voor de Statistiek, 1983; Schraven, 1984).[1]

Holland's diversity is not only from without but also from within. Many different dialects, not accents, are spoken throughout Holland's 11 provinces. Some of the dialects are so pronounced that subtitles must be used when individuals are interviewed on national television! Then there are the Frisians with their own language, literature, and at one time, their own liberation movement.

Not to be overlooked is Holland's religious diversity. Approximately, 31% are Catholic, 25% are Protestant (mainly Calvinists), and 42% have no church affiliation (Galjaard, 1981:202). As we shall see later, religious affiliation was, until recently, central to the organization of Dutch social, political and economic life including the delivery of health and human services. Catholics are concentrated ''south of the rivers'' i.e., the Rhine and Maas Rivers, while Protestants are concentrated in the north.

Size of Disabled Population

It is estimated that as of 1981, some 1.2 million or 9.0% of the Dutch population 5 years of age and over have a *physical* disability because of a limitation in mobility or personal care; or because of a communication or sensory impairment. This estimate of the prevalence of physical disability takes into account the aging of the population since the last survey of physical disability was conducted in 1971. That survey, involving 75,000 respondents, indicated that about 1.0 million persons or 8.7% of the Dutch population had a physical disability (Special Commission on Policy on the Handicapped, n.d.: 147-148; de Kleijn-de Vrankrijker, 1976). The main concern of the monograph is the several thousand persons between 18 and 64 years of age who require daily assistance with their personal care needs.[2]

THE ECONOMIC CONTEXT

The range of services now available to disabled persons would not have been possible without Holland's tremendous postwar economic recovery. This section will briefly recount the scope of that recovery and its impact on the development of Holland's substantial health and welfare system in which disabled persons participate.

The scope of Holland's postwar recover cannot be appreciated without a brief mention of earlier economic events. For the Netherlands, the depression of the 1930's was deeper and longer than for most other West European

---

1. *Some estimate that there are up to 500,000 persons of Surinamese origin living in the Netherlands. The conflicting estimates arise from the fact that many have Dutch citizenship and are not counted as Surinamese.*

2. *The Netherlands does not conduct an ongoing health and disability survey comparable to the annual Health Interview Survey conducted in the United States by the National Center for Health Statistics. The data presented here are the most recent available.*

countries. Holland's economic situation worsened in World War II: Holland lost 55% of its productive capacity in transport and communications because of German bombing and other war-related activities; ran up a huge national debt; and suffered staggering losses of income during the German occupation. During the final stages of the war, consumption had fallen well below subsistence (Klein, 1980). The economic dislocations precipitated by the depression and the war led thousands to immigrate to North America, Australia, and New Zealand.

In the immediate post-war period, the Netherlands was saddled with a 100,000-man colonial army half way around the globe in Indonesia (which gained its independence in 1949) and was hit with disastrous flooding in 1953 in which thousands drowned (de Wolff and Driehuis. 1980). The flooding also prompted one of the largest public works projects in history, known as the Delta Works, in an effort to prevent future disasters arising from Holland's vulnerability to the sea.

Despite all of these dislocations, the Netherlands rapidly reindustrialized itself to become one of the most productive economies in the world. An important factor in the drive for economic modernization was the redevelopment and expansion of the Rotterdam harbor into the world's busiest port today. Throughout the post war period, labor productivity increased dramatically. Increases in real wages followed. Even in the 1970's, labor productivity in manufacturing continued to rise (11.6% in 1976 alone) while in the United States, with an older capital stock, productivity stagnated or declined (de Wolff and Driehuis, 1980).

One other event in Holland's recent economic history should be noted—the discovery of large natural gas fields in the northern province of Groningen. What had made Holland's economic recovery so remarkable was the fact that the country had virtually no natural resources upon which to build except for its splendid geographical position at the mouth of Europe's most important waterways leading to the industrial heart of the continent. The post war recovery was well underway when, in the late 1950's and early 1960's, large natural gas fields were found. The export of natural gas contributed significantly to Holland's foreign exchange position, but more importantly, it also helped to finance a large and deliberate expansion of the public sector. Moreover, the general rise in oil prices starting with the 1973 oil embargo added significantly to government revenues from natural gas sales abroad (Lubbers and Lemchert, 1980).

The year 1973 also ushered in the center-left coalition government of Prime Minister Joop den Uyl (1973-78) and with it a significant shift in economic priorities. For 25 years since the war the Dutch had focused on investment, capital formation, and the rebuilding of their economy. If one adds the war years and the depression years, it could be said that the Dutch had experienced 45 years of deferred living. Now with their economic survival assurred, the Dutch began to turn their attention to issues of income distribution and social welfare. It was time to enjoy the fruits of their hard work and new-found prosperity. Moreover, natural gas exports guaranteed the financing of an expanded welfare state. It was during this period that the public sector increased to over 50% of the country's net national income.

Disabled persons were among the main beneficiaries of this expansion. As will be described in greater detail elsewhere, new legislation was introduced and eligibility for health and disability income benefits was substantially liberalized as were fringe benefits for those in the labor force. The new social policy also reflected a growing national consensus that all elements should share more equitably in the nation's economic prosperity. Today, with unemployment rates 10 percentage points higher than 10 years ago and, more importantly, with deficit spending amounting to 11% of the nation's gross national product, the Netherlands is economically less confident. The nation is struggling to determine whether it can still afford the welfare state in its present form, and the social benefits to which it has become accustomed. This state of affairs was brought into sharp relief when government employees staged a nationwide strike in November of 1983 to protest a proposed 3% reduction in government salaries and benefits that had already failed to keep pace with recent inflation. As we will observe later, disabled persons have not been spared the effects of "cutback government." The question remains whether the Dutch will be as magnanimous toward its disabled citizenry in economic adversity as it has been in economic prosperity.

THE SOCIAL CONTEXT

Central to the understanding of Dutch society is the history of "confessionalization" whereby many social institutions were—and still are—organized along "confessional" or religious lines. Historically, confessionalization has its roots in the 16th century when Holland's long struggle with Spain left Holland divided into two opposing groups, Protestants and Catholics. Despite their mutual hostility, both groups had to find a way to coexist and eventually reach some type of accommodation at the national level. Over many years, both groups developed their own network of social institutions—schools, trade unions, hospitals, welfare agencies, newspapers, broadcasting organizations, and political parties. Not to be overlooked in this all-too-brief history was the development of nonreligious groups with their corollary institutions.

Eventually, this segmentation of Dutch society came to be conceptualized as *verzuiling* or "pillarization" meaning that the overall social system was supported by the various segments or pillars (*zuilen*) that were independent but mutually supportive. In 1917, *verzuiling* or pillarization gained strength when, at the urging of various religious parties, Parliament adopted a law requiring government to subsidize the schools and universities of different religious groups. It was then only a matter of time that government would also subsidize other activities under the control of each *zuil* or religious group.

To catch the flavor of *verzuiling* in its extreme, one might cite the words of van den Berg and Molleman (1975) who write: "Membership in the Catholic swimming club was almost as important as belief in the resurrection."

Closely related to the concept of *verzuiling* is the principle of "subsidiarity," the idea that a function in society (e.g., providing services to persons with disabilities) should be delegated to the lowest social unit capable of carrying out the task, whether it be an individual, the family, or a voluntary agency within a *zuil*. It was the responsibility of each *zuil* to foster the development of voluntary agencies to meet the health and welfare needs of its membership. In the case of services rendered by the public sector, responsibility should be delegated to the lowest level of local and provincial government possible.

The responsibility to develop voluntary organizations became known as the principle of *particulier initiatief* or "private initiative."[3] Today, *particulier initiatief* agencies are commonly referred to as PI agencies or PI's for short. Although often subsidized by government, the principle of subsidiarity requires that government interfere as little as possible and that PI's retain their autonomy with respect to the design and management of their service programs. In the two decades following World War II, PI's became the main providers of social services and also, the cornerstone of the service delivery system for persons with disabilities.

Unfortunately, the concepts of *verzuilen* and *particulier initiatief* also led to a tremendous proliferation and duplication of voluntary agencies that was untenable in a country as small as the Netherlands. A case in point is home health services which will also be discussed at greater length in Section IV. Each home health agency had a different colored cross and flag marking its confessional loyalties—a green cross, a white-yellow cross and others. It was not uncommon for different confessionally based home health agencies to exist side-by-side in the same community. By 1962 there were 979 home health and other types of home help agencies in the Netherlands (Brenton, 1982).

By the early 1970's the unabated proliferation of PI agencies among the *zuilen* became something of a national crises. Although the PI system was heavily subsidized, the national government failed to exercise any of the leverage it had by virtue of being the system's underwriter. It was not until the den Uyl government came to power (1973-78) that the PI system came up for serious review as a result of *Knelpuntennota* or "Bottleneck Report." The report sought to redefine the relationship between government and the PI

---

3. *"Private initiative" is not to be confused with the American use of the term which usually refers to free market, profit-making enterprises. The Dutch use of the term refers to nonmarket, nonprofit enterprises organized by religious and nonreligious groups and supported by donations and government subsidies.*

system. It also sought to diminish the power of the many PI umbrella organizations or *koepels* that become a shadow bureaucracy with its own needs for growth, funding, and professional identity.

More than anything, the *knelpuntennota* helped to establish the terms of the debate about the future of Holland's social welfare system. It helped to set a climate in which efforts were undertaken to consolidate portions of the service delivery system. In the case of home help services, for example, the number of agencies declined to 296 in 1975 and to 241 in 1983. The consolidation of the home help industry has also meant that in many instances, confessional loyalties had to be put aside as confessional agencies were merged with one another and with nonconfessional agencies.

These developments parallel the general demise of confessional distinctions in Dutch society. Since the late 1960's and early 1970's, the traditional religious "pillars" of Dutch society have begun to crumble (*ontzuiling*). Religious loyalties have become blurred and less important. In many instances, PI's, begun under religious auspices, no longer have a distinct religious affiliation and in the course of events have also lost their claim to a well-defined religious constituency.

Despite "deconfessionalization," vestiges of the old system survive. Holland's educational system remains significantly confessionalized. There also are many old style confessional social welfare organizations some of which are directed to the needs of disabled persons. The main legacy of the *verzuiling* is the private sponsorship of service agencies. Most residential and IL programs, for example, are organized as private foundations (each known as a *stichting*) that very much embody the spirit of *particulier initiatief*.

THE POLITICAL CONTEXT

The history of confessionalism has also had a strong impact on Holland's political system, an impact that survives to the present both in party politics and in interest group behavior.

Party Politics

Until the recent past, each of the major religious groups had its own political party. Among the major groups, the Catholics had their Catholic Peoples Party or KVP *(Katholieke Volks Partij)*, mainline Protestants or Calvinists had their Anti-Revolutionary Party or ARP,[4] and the more conservative Calvinists had their Christian Historical Union or CHU. Until 1967, these three parties consistently obtained about 50% of the electoral vote in national elections.

Starting in 1967, we see the electoral effects of deconfessionalization

---

4. *The "anti" in the name of the Anti-Revolutionary Party referred to the party's opposition to the values and philosophy of the French Revolution.*

mentioned earlier. People no longer voted along strict confessional lines as they once did. After 10 years of diminished electoral success, the three main religious parties merged in 1977 to form one party known as the Christian Democratic Appeal or CDA which has since captured a little more than one-third of the vote.

At the moment, the Netherlands has more than 20 political parties, 12 of which are represented in Parliament. Several of these parties orginated in the late 1960's as a result of deconfessionalization and depillarization. Only a handful of these parties ever participate in the formation of government. Three of these parties will be mentioned here. First, is the CDA which is widely viewed as the center party in Holland's political system. Second, is the Labor Party or PvdA *(Partij van de Arbeid)* which is viewed as the leftist party on Holland's political spectrum. Third is the Liberal Party or VVD *(Volkspartij voor Vrijheid en Democratie)* which is viewed as the conservative party.[5]

Since no party has ever gained a majority vote, the Netherlands has had an endless succession of coalition governments. All coalition governments tend to be either center-left or center-right governments with the center party, meaning the CDA, participating as the permanent swing party. This alignment of parties has guaranteed the CDA, Holland's confessional party, some role in the government. It has also guaranteed the survival of Holland's confessional past in the formation of public policy.

However, it is the Labor Party, not the CDA, that has been Holland's largest vote-getter in recent years, routinely obtaining 30 to 40% of the vote. Because of its position in Holland's political spectrum, the Labor Party's vote-getting ability does not guarantee it a role in the government. Often it has been politically more advantageous for the Labor Party to serve as the lead opposition party.

Public policy with respect to persons with disabilities has shifted with changes in coalition governments. In the mid 1970's, the rise of a center-left government in times of economic prosperity (fueled by the sales of natural gas) led to a general expansion and liberalization of disability benefits. Conversely, in the early 1980's, the rise of a center-right government in times of severe economic recession has led to cutbacks in disability benefits.

Interest Group Politics

For all its visibility, party politics is perhaps less significant than interest

---

5. *The label "liberal" in the context of Dutch and European politics has almost the opposite meaning that is has in the United States. In Dutch and European politics, the label "liberal" has some affiity with the American term, "liberterian," although liberals in the Netherlands are neither as fiercely individualistic nor as aggressively capitalistic as their libertarian counterparts in the United States. Compared to American politics, Dutch liberals are the champions of individual rights (much like liberal Democrats in the United States) and advocates of limited government intervention in the market economy (much like mainline Republicans).*

group politics in shaping public policies affecting persons with disabilities in the Netherlands. Like party politics, interest group politics has its roots in, and owes much of its legitimacy to, Holland's religious past.

Interest group politics has a very pejorative connotation in the United States. It creates the image of self-centered special interests feeding out of the public trough. Moreover, interest groups are often thought to distort the public policy decision making process in ways that are inconsistent with the ''public interest'' usually defined as something greater than the sum of all the parts represented by special interests groups.[6]

Although the self-interests of each group cannot be ignored, the Dutch have had a much different experience with interest groups. Interest group politics in the Netherlands is more formalized and institutionalized than in the United States. In the Dutch political system, interest groups are not chaffing at the fringes of the policy making process but are formally consulted and brought into the decision making process itself. Representatives of employer groups, employee groups, government agencies, provider groups, consumer groups, and others are expected to thrash out a consensus that is later ratified by Parliament. In this system, government is not so much an initiator of policy as it is a ratifier of policy.

To describe this system, Dutch and European political scientists (de Beus and van den Doel, 1980; Schmitter, 1974; Lijphart, 1977; Jordan and Richardson, 1983) use terms such as ''corporatism'' and ''neo-corporatism.'' In this system, certain entities or groups are recognized as the only legitimate spokespeople for certain interests. According to Schmitter (1974), such groups are granted a *de facto* license and monopoly to represent a category of interests. In exchange for this license or representational monopoly, groups are expected to exercise a measure of restraint and to abide by the consensus that emerges from the process.

Although characteristic of many Western parliamentary democracies, the corporatist model of interest group politics is particularly strong in the Netherlands. The corporatist approach owes much of its strength to the history of *verzuiling* and the practice of *particulier initiatief* introduced earlier. The corporatist approach in Dutch society helped to establish a long history of formalized consultation and mutual accommodation across confes-

---

6. *Some American political scientists have advanced a more positive view of interest groups in American politics. According to this view, the political process is comprised of atomistically small groups competing with each other in trying to shape policy outcomes. No single interest group is large enough to determine the outcome. When interest groups get large or form coalitions, countervailing groups and coalitions tend to form. Because no group can dictate the outcome, groups must compromise. Oscillations around a given issue are fairly narrow, always tending toward some equilibrium. That equilibrium is considered to be the embodiment of the public interest. Such a system, much like the perfectly competitive market, is said to be self-regulating and inherently stable. This view of interest group politics has been criticized for ignoring the disparate economic advantages that different groups bring to the bargaining and decision making process (Schattschneider, 1975; DeJong, 1979).*

sional lines and between socio-economic groups such as employer and employee groups, professional and consumer groups, and the like. Moreover, the identity of *particulier initiatief* agencies or PI's as independent and autonomous required government to negotiate rather than supervise the administration of many publicly funded health and human services. Over the years many PI's have organized themselves into an extensive labyrinth of umbrella organizations know as *koepels* and *koepeltjes* which in many instances have been recognized by government as the formal bargaining agent in developing policy in the corporatist system.

The locus of bargaining, negotiation, and consultation is usually a council, an advisory body, an interministerial committee, or some other body in which persons from government, the private sector, and other affected groups are represented. There are now hundreds of such quasi-governmental bodies shaping public policy in the Netherlands.

This system is not without its detractors. Many view the system as not only unwieldy but as an extra-parliamentary government that is usurping the powers of representative government usually ascribed to parliament. It has been criticized as an invisible subterranean government, an ungovernable "twilight state," where the distinction between public and private sectors becomes blurred and where accountability is limited to the constituent groups represented in the process.

Its positive features should not be overlooked. The frequent use of consultation insures that affected groups and differing viewpoints will not be overlooked. Moreover, the process has helped to insure a high level of consensus in Dutch society on most public policy issues. All affected parties feel they have participated in the decision making process and as a result feel they have a stake in the outcome. This state of affairs may also account for the high degree of social cohesion and the lack of social friction on many otherwise prickly social and economic issues.

To illustrate how this extra-parliamentary system operates in the case of policy issues affecting disabled persons, one might consider the composition and function of the Interministerial Steering Group on Rehabilitation Policy established in 1970. From the public sector, the Steering Group is comprised of representatives from several ministries of which the Ministry of Welfare, Public Health & Culture serves as the lead or coordinating ministry.[7] From the private sector, the Steering Committee is comprised of representatives from groups such as the Dutch Rehabilitation Association or NVR *(Nederlandse Verenigingen voor Revalidatie)* and, until recently, the National Organization for the Care of the Mentally Retarded or NOZ.

Both the NVR and NOZ are examples of umbrella groups or *koepels* men-

---

7. *The other ministries include Social Affairs & Employment; Education & Science; Housing, Land Use Planning, & Environmental Policy; and Defense. The Steering Group is also comprised of* ad hoc *members and observers from other ministries and from other steering groups.*

tioned earlier. The Steering Group pretty much regards these two umbrella organizations as the most appropriate groups with which to discuss matters related to the needs of disabled persons:

> Only on very rare occasions do talks take place between the Interministerial Steering Group and non-umbrella organizations, one reason being that this might undermine the position of the umbrella organizations (Interministerial Steering Group on Rehabilitation Policy, 1981:95).

This statement clearly indicates the extent to which preference is given to consultation with umbrella groups which serve as bargaining agents for their constituent organizations. It is also interesting to note that, in times past, questions have been raised as to whether constituent member organizations of umbrella groups could be admitted as observers to meetings of the Interministerial Steering Group. The prevailing view of the Interministerial Steering Group (1981:96) is that such participation would compromise the channels of communication between public and private sectors in shaping disability policy.

The workings of the Interministerial Steering Committee clearly illustrate how interest group politics in the Netherlands is more institutionalized and built into the corporate structure of public policy making than in the United States. Interest groups are not free to enter the bargaining process except through the channel of their respective umbrella organizations. In the United States, smaller interest groups may be a part of a larger national umbrella organization but are never precluded from registering their views in testimony before Congress or in formally voicing their opinions to federal officials as, for example, in the 60-day review period for new federal regulations.

A closer look at the NVR and several related organizations will also give us a better understanding of interest group politics and the larger community of interests that shape portions of disability policy in the Netherlands.

The NVR is comprised of about 150 organizations and groups, mainly service providers such as institutions for sensory impaired persons, rehabilitation centers, professional groups, residential care providers, and others. NVR's relationship with the consumer community has been a strained one. During the early and mid 1970's consumer representation on NVR's board of directors increased from 2 to 6 voting members out of a total of 30 voting members, still leaving consumer groups with only 20% of the vote.

In 1977, the various consumer groups broke away from the NVR to form the Council of Dutch Disabled or GR *(Nederlandse Gehandicaptenraad)*. The GR's closest counterpart in the United States would be ACCD, the American Coalition of Citizens with Disabilities. The GR is composed of 37 consumer groups some of which represent specific disabling conditions while others are more cross-disability in character. Cross-disability groups are commonly known as general disability organizations and in a couple of instances have roots in Holland's confessionalized past. Two of these groups will be mentioned here: First is the General Dutch Disability Alliance or ANIB *(Algenene Nederlandse Invalid Bond),* a nonconfessional group comprised of 27,000 individuals. And second is the Organization of the Disabled in the Netherlands or GON *(Gehandicapten Organatie van Nederland)* which used to be the Catholic disability group.

The departure of the GR from the NVR clearly illustrates how consumer-provider antagonisms have replaced the religious antagonisms that were characteristic of Holland's more confessionalized past. The NVR has become the representative for the organized supply side of "the market" while the GR has become the organized demand side of the "market."

The GR's departure from the NVR resulted in two umbrella organizations rather than one trying to speak for the needs of disabled persons. Given the Dutch tradition of having only one umbrella organization within a particular policy area, the two umbrella organizations, the NVR and the GR, formed a new super umbrella organization in 1980 known as the National Organization for Disability Policy or NOG *(Nationaal Orgaan Gehandicapten-beleid)* in which both constituent organizations, the NVR and the GR, have equal representation. At present, there is a major struggle within the NOG. GR representatives believe that the GR should be the sole official consultative group on national policy matters and that the NVR's role should simply be an advisory one. As of this writing, the outcome of this struggle remains to be seen. It is widely thought that the GR will become the only or leading group to speak on disability issues and that the NVR will have a diminished role or even go out of existence. The outcome of this struggle will also determine who will be represented on national policy making groups such as the Interministerial Steering Committee on Rehabilitation Policy.

This struggle reflects the increasing assertiveness of disabled persons in Dutch society. It also reflects the idea that the interests of disabled persons should not be mediated through provider-based organizations.

The struggle between provider and consumer interests is also reflected in Holland's residential & IL system. For example, the various large and small residential centers introduced in Section I are represented in the Dutch Federation of Service Centers for the Physically Disabled *(Nederlandse Federatie van Voorzieningscentra voor Lichamelijk Gehandicapten),* a member organization within the NVR. However, the residents within the various living centers are persons with disabilities whose loyalties in many cases are with consumer organizations such as the GR.

I have used the Interministerial Steering Committee and its constituent groups to illustrate the character of interest group politics. However, the Interministerial Steering Group on Rehabilitation Policy is not the only arena in which disability policy is made. Disability umbrella organizations also participate on other councils and steering committees. For example, the GR is represented on the Health Insurance Council or ZFR *(Ziekenfondsraad)* which has much to say about health insurance and other in-kind benefits of interest to disabled persons. This phenomenon illustrates the strategy of interest groups to ''penetrate'' as many policy making entities as possible. The GR has not, however, penetrated the Social Security Council or SVR *(Sociale Verzekeringsraad)*. The SVR is one of the more important councils since it has much to say about the scope of income benefits available to disabled persons. The council is still a stronghold of more traditional corporatism since participation is limited to employer and employee groups (in addition to the ''crown members'' who serve as governmentally appointed experts). The various disability related income and in-kind benefits supervised by the SVR and the ZFR will be discussed in the next section.

III THE SOCIAL & HEALTH INSURANCE SYSTEM FOR DISABLED PERSONS

To a much larger extent than in the United States, services that enable disabled persons to live independently, are financed through Holland's social and health insurance system. In the United States, services such as specially adapted private transportation, adapted housing, and attendant care are often financed through ''ad hoc'' programs that are independent of, or at the fringes of, American social and health insurance systems. One example of an ad hoc program is the federal-state vocational rehabilitation system. By contrast, many services paid through the American vocational rehabilitation program are routinely paid through Holland's mainline entitlement programs. As a result, the services that enable disabled persons to live independently are more widely viewed as entitlements in the Netherlands than in the United States.

Thus, critical to the understanding of independent living in the Netherlands is some knowledge of Holland's (1) major social insurance programs, and (2) major health insurance and long-term care funding programs as they apply to persons with disabilities.[1] In addition special attention will be given to the provision of in-kind benefits (e.g., equipment and adaptations) that are of special interest to persons with severe self-care limitations. Altogether, 6 programs will be introduced: 4 social insurance programs and 2 health-related programs. These 6 programs will be referenced with considerable frequency in the next section when we discuss the various residential and IL models in some detail.

MAJOR SOCIAL INSURANCE PROGRAMS

Before describing the various social insurance programs, we must consider a peculiarity of Dutch social and economic life known as ''trade associations'' which have a major role in the administration of social insurance benefits.

Trade Associations

In the Netherlands, a disabled person's social insurance benefits do not ordinarily come from a government source. Instead a person's benefits come via his or her ''membership'' in one of Holland's 26 ''trade associations'' or *bedrijfsverenigingen*. These trade associations are not trade unions but rather groupings of industries and occupations.[2] Trade associations collect

---

1. The principal sources of information for this section include Vereniging van Raden van Arbeid (1984) [commonly known as de Kleine Gids]; Emanuel, Halberstadt, and Petersen (1980); SZW (1982 & 1984); and many interviewees.
2. Examples of trade associations include trade associations for agriculture, dairy industry, textile industry, chemical industry, bakers, meat and butcher industry, lodging and restaurant industry, and the trade association for banking, insurance, wholesalers, and self-employed professionals.

the funds they need by levying social premiums on both employers and employees.

The boards of trade associations are comprised of representatives from
employer organizations and trade unions within a given "branch of industry." Trade associations are a clear example of the "do-it-yourself" principle
of subsidiarity and the concept of corporatism discussed in Section II. Each
trade association operates fairly independently but within a national legal
framework that provides for similar eligibility criteria and a similar package
of social insurance benefits.

An important organization in the lives of many disabled persons is the
Joint Medical Service or GMD (*Gemeenschappelijke Medische Dienst*) which
advises the trade associations regarding the medical and vocational merits of
a person's application for disability benefits. The GMD employs a few hun-
dred "social insurance" physicians scattered in 27 district offices. The GMD
not only advises regarding a person's eligibility for income benefits but also a
person's need for in-kind benefits such as assistive devices, in-home adaptations, an accessible automobile, and attendant care. The trade associations
generally follow the advice of the GMD in these matters. In a sense, the GMD
offers a "one-stop" evaluation system for most of a disabled person's IL needs.

Policy coordination across all 26 trade associations with respect to social
insurance is the formal responsibility of the Social Insurance Council or the
SVR (*Sociale Verzekeringsraad*) introduced in Section II. In practice, most
coordination is done by the Federation of Trade Associations.

With this brief introduction to trade associations, we are now prepared
to consider each of the major social insurance programs as they pertain to
persons with severe disabilities.

Sickness Benefit Act (ZW)

The Sickness Benefit Act or ZW (*Ziektewet*) provides cash benefits during a worker's first year of illness or disability. This wage-replacement program starts on the third day of absence from work. The legal minimum
benefit is set at 80% of one's regular earnings. In many cases, depending on
the trade association to which a person belongs, employers will supplement
this package by (1) providing benefits after the first day of absence from work
and (2) by augmenting benefits to 100% of one's regular earnings.

Medical screening for sickness benefits is not conducted by the GMD but
by company-retained physicians, family physicians, or by physicians and
"lay controllers" employed by trade associations.

Work Disability Insurance Act (WAO)

The Work Disability Insurance Act or WAO (*Wet op de Arbeidsongeschikheidsverzekering*) picks up where the ZW leaves off, i.e., it becomes
effective when a person has been ill or disabled for more than one year and is
no longer eligible for ZW benefits. The WAO is targeted to working age per-

sons. Its benefits are based on (1) previous earnings and (2) degree of disability. The maximum benefit is 80% of previous earning and scaled downward depending on the degree of disability. In no case is the benefit less than the legal minimum wage which varies with age and the employment status of the spouse.[3]

The American counterpart to the WAO is the SSDI (Social Security Disability Insurance) program. The WAO is, however, different from the SSDI program in 2 important respects:

First, the WAO considers the claimant's degree of disability whereas a SSDI claimant must be found either disabled or not disabled. Under the WAO program, a person must be only 15% disabled to qualify for some benefits. Degrees of disability are hard to establish on purely medical grounds. Instead, degree of disability is determined by the amount of income foregone resulting from a reduced capacity to do one's usual work or other work taking into account a person's previous training and work experience. The lack of suitable alternative employment—even if attributable to poor labor market conditions—can qualify a person for a 100% degree of disability.

Second, WAO benefit levels are not based on a person's work history (extended over 5 years or so as in the United States), but on what a person would have earned in his former occupation had he or she not become disabled— usually defined as the claimant's most recent earnings. Thus, the WAO is an "end-wage" system, not an "average wage" system as is the SSDI program.[4]

As in the case of the ZW mentioned above, the WAO is administered through Holland's network of trade associations. All claims for WAO benefits are reviewed by the GMD to determine degree of disability. In most instances, the trade association will accept the findings of the GMD.

Public employees, railway workers, and military personnel do not participate in the WAO program but have their own disability insurance programs which have similar eligibility criteria and benefit levels.

General Work Disability Act (AAW)

The General Work Disability Act or AAW (*Algemene Arbeidsonge-schikheids Wet*) is the companion program to the WAO. It provides a general or flat rate disability benefit above which WAO benefits are paid if a person's earnings in the previous year exceeded the minimum wage upon which AAW benefits are computed. The AAW program also covers groups not covered by the WAO such as those who are self-employed and those who have never

---

3. *Unlike the United States, European countries are more prone to take into account the employment status of the spouse in their respective tax and social insurance policies. At the risk of oversimplification, a second income is often viewed as a "luxury." In the Netherlands, the second income is taxed more heavily than the first income and is also considered when computing a person's legal minimum wage and disability benefits.*

4. *Because of the high cost associated with Holland's disability system, it is likely that it will eventually become more of an "average wage" system.*

worked because their disability began in childhood.

In a sense, the AAW program is somewhat like the American Supplemental Security Income (SSI) program. Both the AAW and SSI programs provide a flat minimum disability income benefit. Beyond this common feature, the AAW and SSI programs differ: most importantly, unlike SSI, AAW benefits are based on degree of disability as in the WAO program.[5]

As in the American SSDI and SSI programs, a person can have dual entitlement, i.e., receive benefits from both the WAO and AAW programs. However, dual entitlement serves different functions in the American and Dutch systems. In the American system, the SSI program serves to supplement the SSDI program when SSDI benefits (based on previous earnings) are below the SSI payment level. In the Dutch system, it is the other way around: the WAO program serves to supplement the AAW benefit when previous earnings warrant. Thus, all WAO beneficiaries also receive an AAW benefit that serves as a built-in floor. The WAO benefit is only provided to the extent to which it exceeds the AAW benefit.

From the perspective of independent living, a significant feature of the AAW program is its ability to also fund in-kind services and equipment such as durable medical equipment (e.g., wheelchairs), technical aids (e.g., communication devices), home modifications, automobile adaptations, and attendant care. This feature of the AAW program will be discussed at greater length in a later part of this section.

General Assistance Act (ABW)

Those who do not qualify for any of the programs mentioned above, and have no other means of support, are picked up under Holland's "safety net" program known as the General Assistance Act or ABW (*Algemene Bijstandswet*).[6] The ABW is not a social insurance program and is not administered through Holland's system of trade associations but instead through municipalities under the supervision of the Ministry of Social Affairs and Employment.

HEALTH INSURANCE & LONG-TERM CARE FUNDING

In addition to the role of cash income transfer programs, we must also consider the role of Holland's health care financing system which has had a substantial impact upon services and alternatives available to disabled persons. Two health-related financing programs are discussed below: (1) The Sickness Fund Law and (2) the General Exceptional Medical Expenses Act.

---

5. *To qualify for AAW benefits, a person must be at least 25% disabled, not just 15% as in the WAO program.*

6. *A case in point would be a working age person who was not eligible for WAO or AAW benefits because he or she was not gainfully employed (but was studying or keeping house) when the disabling event occurred.*

Sickness Fund Law (ZFW)

The Sickness Fund Law or ZFW (*Ziekenfondswet*) is Holland's basic health insurance program in which about 75% of the population participates. The ZFW provides payment for most customary medical expenses, both in-patient and outpatient. From the perspective of independent living, the ZFW is important because it is an important source of funding for durable medical equipment and other services during a person's first year of disablement.

General Exceptional Medical Expenses Act (AWBZ)

The General Exceptional Medical Expenses Act or AWBZ (*Algemene Wet Bijzondere Ziektekosten*) is Holland's catastrophic health insurance and long-term care funding program covering the entire population. The AWBZ is one of the most important programs in the lives of disabled persons. It pays for health and social services required beyond the acute phase of care including medical rehabilitation services, durable medical equipment, and nursing home care. As a long-term care funding program, the AWBZ underwrites most of the residential care system introduced earlier in this monograph. As will be seen later, the AWBZ is also the main funding source for community-based home health services, a source of assistance for those persons seeking to live apart from an organized housing program.

Administration and Supervision

These 2 programs are not administered through Holland's network of trade associations but through about 60 ''sickness funds'' that have evolved along confessional, political, and regional lines. The sickness funds are supervised by the Health Insurance Council or ZFR (*Ziekenfondsraad*) which also provides policy direction for the ZFW and AWBZ programs. The ZFR (briefly mentioned in Section II) is one of Holland's more important consultative bodies and is another example of ''corporatist'' politics. The ZFR includes representation from employer groups, employee groups, sickness funds, physician groups, ''crown members,'' and consumer groups such as the Dutch Handicapped Council or GR (introduced in Section II).

IN-KIND BENEFITS AND THE ROLE OF THE GMD

As indicated on several occasions, Holland's social insurance programs are more than cash transfer programs. They also provide in-kind benefits such as durable medical equipment, technical aids, home modifications, adapted automobiles, attendant care, and the like. Since the provision of in-kind benefits is a matter that cuts across several social and health insurance programs and is so vital to a person's ability to live independently, the subject of in-kind benefits is given separate consideration here.

At the risk of overgeneralizing, the division of responsibility for the funding of nonresidential in-kind benefits is as follows: The ZFW will pay for special equipment (e.g., wheelchairs) during the acute phase of care; the AWBZ will pay for special equipment and adaptations during the rehabilitation phase of care (and if an individual is discharged to a long-term care facility); and the AAW will pay for the equipment, adaptations, and services needed during the post rehabilitation or IL phase of a disabled person's life. Concurrent with the AAW's funding role is the role of the Ministry of Housing (VROM) in funding home modifications for persons living independently.

In later sections of this monograph we will observe some exceptions to this pattern of funding as in the case of ABWZ-funded home health services for those living in their own homes apart from an organized housing program.

The Strategic Role of the AAW

Of the various sources of funding for in-kind benefits, the AAW is the most important for at least 3 reasons:

First, the AAW covers nearly all disabled persons between 18 and 65 years of age. As noted earlier, the AAW is Holland's general disability law that provides a basic payment both to those who receive WAO cash benefits as well as most of those with insufficient earnings to qualify for WAO cash benefits. In addition, the AAW covers other groups not protected by the WAO program including public employees (who receive AAW benefits as a floor for their own disability insurance program), the self-employed, part-time workers, domestic workers, and persons whose disability began prior to their working years. Thus, the scope of the AAW's eligibility criteria guarantees that most disabled persons will be covered by the AAW.[7]

Second, the AAW provides broad authority for the financing of in-kind benefits. The statute authorizes the provision of in-kind benefits when they are directed to one or both of two goals: (1) to help an individual become gainfully employed or (2) to help an individual live more independently. Either of these two goals can be invoked to secure durable medical equipment (e.g., wheelchairs), adaptive devices, accessible private transportation, in-home assistance, and the like.

Third, the AAW serves as a back-up program for in-kind benefits that, in some instances, cannot be acquired through the ZFW or AWBZ. The AAW will pay for durable medical equipment and technical aids if the requested item is not on the ZFW list or the AWBZ list of approved items. The ZFW and AWBZ lists are politicized documents since third party reimbursement is so essential to the marketing of devices by vendors and manufacturers. Items not yet on the ZFW or AWBZ lists, because they are new or unconventional, can almost always be paid by the AAW.

Aside from any contributions made by the AWBZ, the AAW is virtually the sole source of funding for most IL needs during the post-hospital period.

---

7. *It should also be mentioned that persons can sometimes qualify for AAW-funded in-kind benefits without qualifying for AAW cash benefits.*

In a single source of funding system, important trade-offs can be thoughtfully considered. For example, an investment in adapted equipment can reduce the need for attendant care and thus save costs over the long run. Such trade-offs are virtually impossible in the United States where in-kind benefits, such as those financed by the AAW, must be obtained from a myriad of agencies, each with separate funding sources, eligibility requirements, and evaluation procedures. In the American system, each agency manager has the incentive to remain the payor of last resort and to let another agency or funding source assume the costs of special needs. The Dutch have their share of "buck-passing" problems but they are minor compared to those found in the United States.

Also important to note is the fact that, unlike its companion program in the United States (the SSI program mentioned earlier), the AAW is both a cash benefit program and an in-kind benefit program. By making in-kind benefits an inherent part of a cash entitlement program, the Dutch have conferred a quasi-entitlement status to the acquisition of IL-related in-kind benefits. Such a status insures a high level of support for equipment and services needed to live independently.

The Strategic Role of the GMD

Not to be overlooked is the important role of the GMD in evaluating a person's need for AAW-funded in-kind benefits in addition to GMD's role in evaluating a person's medical and vocational status when applying for WAO and AAW cash benefits. In some cases the need for in-kind benefits may be delegated to a service provider such as a home health agency or a Fokus project but it remains the responsibility of the GMD to make final recommendations to the relevant trade associations.[8]

The GMD also works closely with the Ministry of Housing (VROM) which has been delegated responsibility for funding home modifications—one item not covered by the AAW in-kind benefits package.[9] Although the Ministry of Housing represents another funding source, the involvement of the GMD assures some level of coordination in addressing a person's IL needs across administrative boundaries.[10]

The extent of the GMD's evaluation in reviewing a person's need for in-

---

8. *The GMD also evaluates the need for home modifications and in-home assistance on behalf of the Ministry of Welfare, Public Health, and Culture for those individuals who do not qualify for AAW benefits and instead are covered by Holland's safety net program, ABW.*

9. *The Ministry of Housing funds about f70 million ($28 million) of home modifications per year. The Ministry of Housing will subsidize the total cost of modifications up to f6.000 ($2,400) and will subsidize the interest on loans used to finance modifications costing more than f6.000.*

10. *In administering the home modifications program, the Ministry of Housing addresses mainly the technical aspects of the modifications while the GMD addresses the medical and social aspects. This arrangement has sometimes provoked criticism since the involvement of more than one agency prolongs the evaluation and approval process.*

kind assistance varies considerably depending, in part, upon the severity of a person's disability. The role of the GMD is not a cursory one as, for example, in the case of a newly spinal cord injured person. While the person is still in medical rehabilitation, the GMD is notified of the possible need for special equipment or assistance. A team of GMD experts is formed (a physician, a vocational rehabilitation counselor, and a legal advisor) to work with the hospital-based rehabilitation team to begin discharge planning. At least one person from the 3-person GMD team meets with the hospital team every 2 weeks. In addition, each local GMD office has a technical aids expert who is consulted in determining the most appropriate and economical solution in coping with architectural barriers in the home or a related problem. The purpose in each case is to facilitate a smooth transition from hospital to home life (or whatever the discharge goal may happen to be) by taking into account the full range of equipment and services needed to live independently. The extent to which the GMD actually follows this needs assessment strategy is difficult to ascertain. However, it is a strategy designed to provide resources in a timely fashion to facilitate reintegration and the resumption of one's customary social role.

Unfortunately, the GMD is not always notified of special needs in less dramatic cases. All too often, persons become accustomed to the disabled role when timely intervention such as a work site modification, based on a GMD evaluation, could lead to the maintenance of a more productive lifestyle. Mandatory reporting, for example, during the 13th week of ZW benefits has not proved to be workable.

In any event, the GMD's role is an intriguing one. In addition to offering a one-stop evaluation system for in-kind benefits, it insures a relatively high degree of service planning and coordination that helps to minimize the amount of ''buck passing'' between funding sources that might otherwise occur.

COST AND UTILIZATION

Holland's disability-related social insurance programs are costly. In 1983, the Netherlands spent an estimated f30.7 billion ($12.2 billion) for 4 of the main disability-related social and health insurance programs reviewed here —ZW, WAO, AAW, and AWBZ (see table 3-1).[11] These cost figures do not include expenditures from general revenues for programs such as the ABW nor do they include some of the government contributions made on behalf of public employees for their disability insurance programs.

These 4 main disability-related insurance programs—ZW, WAO, AAW, and AWBZ—are financed with premiums paid by employers and employees to the various disability insurance funds (through their respective trade asso-

---

11. *Most ZW expenditures should be viewed as income replacement expenditures for short-term illness.*

ciations) and to the various sickness funds. As of January 1984, the premiums for these 4 programs amounted to 35.35% of income above the minimum wage up to f62.850 ($25,140) of income per year (see Table 3-2).

Present day costs represent a considerably higher percentage of Holland's gross domestic product (GDP) than a decade or two ago. Emanuel et al. (1980) report that the cost of disability-related insurance programs rose from 2.7% of GDP in 1963 to 7.6% of GDP in 1978. The 4 main disability-related insurance programs—ZW, WAO, AAW, and AWBZ—consumed 9.0% of GDP in 1983.

This growth parallels the growth of (1) Holland's public social and health insurance programs in general and (2) Holland's overall public sector over the last 20 years. Holland's public social and health insurance programs have grown from 10.7% of GDP in 1963 to 23.7% of GDP in 1983. During this same time period, Holland's overall public sector has grown from 37.3% of GDP in 1963 to about 59.0% of GDP in 1983.[12] To a large extent, this growth has been deliberate and planned in response to a significant shift in national priorities noted earlier in the monograph.

As of January 1984, 730,000 persons were participating in Holland's 2 most important disability insurance programs, the WAO and AAW. This figure is astounding when one considers the fact that the Netherlands has a population of 14.3 million and a labor force of about 4.0 million.[13] At least three reasons have been given for this high rate of participation: First, only modest amounts of reduced working capacity (15% under the WAO and 25% under the AAW) are required to gain entry into the system. Second, wage-replacement rates of up to 80 to 100% of previous earnings make the receipt of disability income benefits economically attractive and discourage return to work. Third, the economic status of disability insurance beneficiaries is (1) protected through periodic indexing to account for inflation and (2) enhanced through periodic indexing to account for the overall rise in wage rates exclusive of inflation.[14]

It is estimated that at least half of all WAO and AAW beneficiaries are either psychiatrically disabled or have an ailment that is medically nonspe-

---

12. *Cost data were obtained or derived from the following sources: Centraal Planbureau (1982); Emanuel, Halberstadt, & Petersen (1980); OECD (1983); and SZW (1984).*

13. *In the Netherlands, each person in the labor force supports 3.5 persons (him/herself and 2.5 other persons) while, in the United States, each person in the labor force supports 2.2 persons (him/herself and 1.2 other persons). A couple of reasons for these different ratios are worth mentioning. First, the Netherlands has proportionately more persons of retirement age. Second, The Netherlands has proportionately fewer women in its labor force. Compared to the United States, most Dutch women with children, even with school age children, opt not to participate in the labor force. In fact, the Netherlands has one of the lowest labor force participation rates for women in the western industrialized world. This is made possible, in part, by Holland's family allowance program which provides a cash payment for each child in the family.*

14. *However, during this period of declining real wages, beneficiaries will not benefit from this second method of indexing.*

cific such as low-back pain.

Moreover, it is widely assumed by policy experts that Holland's disability insurance system disguises significant amounts of structural unemployment. Holland's relatively liberal eligibility criteria allows one to acquire income protection against structural unemployment under the guise of a disability and thus legitimize one's nonparticipation in the labor force. This is particularly the case with older workers who are displaced by automation but lack the skills needed for alternative employment. For such individuals, disability income is also a way of easing a person into early retirement without significantly disturbing a person's long-term retirement benefits. In a sense, significant portions of Holland's disability insurance programs are *de facto* unemployment insurance and early retirement programs. It is for this reason that Dutch policy experts often cite two unemployment rates: (1) an official unemployment rate and (2) an unofficial unemployment rate that takes into account the unemployment hidden in Holland's disability insurance programs. The latter is sometimes 1.5 times higher than the former.

While necessary to understanding the scope of Holland's disability programs, this macro survey of costs and utilization, in a sense, does a disservice to those persons with very severe disabilities who require IL services—the target group for purposes of this paper. Persons with severe mobility and self-care limitations make up a relatively small proportion of all disability insurance beneficiaries. This is reflected in the fact that the cost and utilization of in-kind benefits, mainly of concern to a limited number of severely disabled beneficiaries, comprise a rising but still very small fraction of all disability insurance benefits. Nevertheless, Holland's disability insurance system constitutes the larger framework in which persons with severe disabilities must cope and acquire the resources needed to live independently. Finally, the future well-being of severely disabled persons in the Netherlands cannot be considered apart from how the current cutback-minded government is seeking to come to terms with the high cost and utilization of the present system. The impact and implications of these cutbacks will be addressed in the context of the various IL alternatives for disabled persons to be discussed in the next 2 sections of this monograph.

Table 3-1
Cost of Disability-related Insurance Programs
(1983)

Program	Guilders (billions)	Dollars[a] (billions)
ZW	f 6.6	$ 2.6
WAO	7.2	2.9
AAW	8.6	3.4
AWBZ	8.3	3.3
Total	f30.7	$12.2

a. 1 dollar = 2.5 guilders
SOURCE: SZW (1984)

Table 3-2
Disability Insurance Premiums (Tax Rates)—January 1984

Program	Premiums (Tax Rates)			Max. Annual Taxable Income	
	Employer	Employee	Total[a]	Guilders	Dollars[b]
ZW	4.80%	1.00%	5.80%	f68.120[c]	$27,298
WAO[a].	1.50	17.60	19.10	68.120[c]	27,258
AAW	6.50	—	6.50	62,850	25,140
AWBZ	3.95	—	3.95	62,850	25,140
TOTAL[a]	16.75	18.60	35.35[a]	62.850	25,140

a. WAO premiums only apply to the interval of income above minimum wage
[f91,00 ($36.40) per day or f23.660 ($9,464) per year assuming 260 working days per year] up to f262,00 ($104.80) per day or f68.120 ($27,248) per
year. Persons earning the minimum wage do not contribute to the WAO
program. Thus the total premiums only apply to the interval above the
minimum income but below the maximums indicated in the table.
b. For purposes of this table, 1 dollar = 2.5 guilders.
c. The maximum taxable income for the ZW and WAO is actually expressed
in daily terms as f262,00 per day. The above annualized figure assumes
260 working days per year.
SOURCE: Vereniging van Raden van Arbeid (1984:77).

IV HOLLAND'S 3-PART RESIDENTIAL & IL SYSTEM

A key characteristic of the Dutch residential care and independent living (IL) system is its emphasis on residential programs and housing projects. Even the services available to an individual under Holland's various social insurance programs are usually made available through a recognized residential program or housing project. Generally speaking, it is more difficult for a disabled person to acquire services as an individual than as a participant in an established program. Even persons living apart from an organized residential program, must rely to a large extent upon organized community-based services.

As mentioned in the introductory section of this monograph, Holland's IL system—if it may rightfully be called that—consists of three main alternatives or models:

    (1) The residential center model (*woonvormen*)

        A. Large residential centers (*grote woonvormen*)

        B. Small residential centers (*kleine woonvormen*)

    (2) The clustered housing model (*Fokus projecten*)

    (3) The independent housing model (*op zich zelf wonen*)

The purpose of this section is to offer an analytic survey of these models, viewing each as part of a much larger system undergoing various degrees of stress in response to competition among the models and in response to funding cutbacks. In the next and final section (Section V), I will try to show that even though elements of Holland's IL system are incongruous with the value and expectations of the American IL movement, the Dutch system has many features that deserve emulation and adaptation to the American context.

THE RESIDENTIAL CENTER MODEL

Holland's system of residential centers consists of 4 large centers accommodating 90 to 400 residents, and 22 smaller centers accommodating 20 to 42 residents. Although a case could be made to consider the larger and smaller residential centers as two different models, their differences are more in scale than in program or in the degree of personal autonomy and privacy they offer to individual residents. Their similarities stem to a large extent from their common funding source, the AWBZ, introduced in Section III as Holland's principal long-term care financing program.

Het Dorp

No discussion about Holland's IL system can begin without mentioning Het Dorp, Holland's largest residential program located on the fringes of Arnhem. Designed to accommodate up to 400 residents, Het Dorp was meant to simulate all the features of a typical autonomous Dutch village community[1]

---

1. *Het Dorp literally means "the Village."*

that would also be frequented by nondisabled persons.

Het Dorp had its beginnings in the early 1960's with a national telethon that, in a matter of days, raised 23 million guilders for "a village" that would be a model of disabled living. Adults opened their pocketbooks and children collected matchbook covers that would be redeemed by local merchants in the form of contributions for Het Dorp.

Today, Het Dorp is a community spread over more than 100 acres of hilly terrain. It is comprised of small individual housing units, work stations, recreational facilities, and a small shopping center not unlike the array of small neighborhood shops to be found in every Dutch village and city. A restaurant and a gas station also help to give Het Dorp the appearance of normality. These facilities are linked through a network of accessible indoor and outdoor passageways.

Het Dorp was Holland's answer to institutionalization. It was thought that a fully accessible and self-contained community with access to the larger Arnhem community would allow disabled persons to manage their own affairs and provide greater contact with the outside world. Today, this social experiment—to which interested foreign observers still make at least one pilgrimage—is often viewed as something of a national embarassment: It is commonly referred to, with shrugged shoulders, as a "disabled ghetto" running counter to the principles of social integration.

Even though it is now viewed with some embarassment, many of Het Dorp's primary features still remain the historic and programmatic point of departure for much of Holland's IL system. Contrary to what many Dutch observers may think, Het Dorp is not just an historical oddity. Many of its prime features have survived into the present among newer and smaller residential centers—for example, the use of centralized attendant care, dependence on AWBZ funding, participation in "social workplaces," giving street names to hallways, and assigning street addresses and private mailboxes to each individual dwelling unit. These features and others are discussed below.

Chief Features of the Residential Center Model

It would be impossible to describe all 4 large and 22 small residential centers. Most residential centers are fairly consistent with respect to the following features: (1) location and physical layout, (2) governance and staffing, (3) attendant care or "ADL assistance," (4) meals, (5) required activities, (6) privacy and sexuality, and (7) financing. However, exceptions do occur. Each of these features are reviewed below.

Location and physical layout. Most residential centers are located in urban areas. Almost all centers are within wheeling distance of a neighborhood-based shopping and service center and therefore are not totally cut off from the community.

A typical residential center is located on one or two floors under one roof with rooms for recreation, communal eating, staff, laundry facilities and the like. Each individual has his or her own living unit. Most are 1-person units; a few are 2-person units to accommodate married persons with disabilities. Most centers are not well-equipped to handle families with children. Hallways are often given street names and each living unit usually has a separate street address to denote individualization and privacy.

A typical living unit consists of one or two bedrooms, a living area, an accessible bathroom, and a kitchen area with adapted but limited cooking and food storage capacity (and perhaps some laundry appliances). The living area often has a large picture window, so common in Dutch homes, overlooking an open outdoor area. This feature as well, is designed to give each individual unit a noninstitutional character.

Governance and staffing. Each residential center is initiated and organized by a foundation or *stichting* with a board of directors and a charter. The foundation is a typical example of private sector initiative or *particulier initiatief* cited in Section II of this monograph. Thus, though heavily subsidized, residential centers are typically private, not governmental, organizations. In some cases, residents and/or staff are represented on the foundation board. Board decisions are delegated to an on site director. While larger residential centers typically have more than one layer of staff, the smaller centers usually have one director and a cadre of attendants known as "ADL assistants." Most residential centers also have a residents (*bewoners*) council with limited powers akin to that of an American college student council.

Attendant care ("ADL assistance"). One of the most persistent features of the entire Dutch system, both in residential centers and in Fokus projects, is the use of centrally stationed, nonuniformed, on-call, ADL assistants. There is some variation among larger and smaller residential centers with respect to ADL assistance.[2]

At Het Dorp, ADL assistants, known as *dogelas*, remain very much in the background and are expected to take a very nondirectional approach to caregiving. At Nieuw Unicum, Holland's second largest residential center (200 residents), ADL assistance is actually provided by a staff of full- and part-time nurses comparable in training to licensed practical nurses (LPNs) in the United States. However, nurses at Nieuw Unicum do not wear uniforms and are expected to perform their duties at the direction of the care recipient. Recipient-direction with respect to his/her own bodily care appears to be highly valued.

Smaller residential centers do not use nurse-trained ADL assistants. A typical smaller residential center will always have a small contingent of ADL assistants (2 to 6 persons) on duty at all times with additional staffing to help

---

2. *ADL assistance is the term most commonly used in the Netherlands and the term that will, for the most part, be used for the balance of this monograph.*

43

during the busier times of the day. ADL assistants can be called by residents with a push of a button that lights a number in the central station area to indicate which resident is requesting service. ADL assistants are not allowed to enter a resident's dwelling unless requested to do so by the resident. Except for part-time staff, ADL assistants work in 8-hour shifts. ADL assistants tend to be younger working age women and are usually paid the minimum wage or higher depending on the length of service. The hiring, firing, and evaluation of ADL assistants is commonly done by a committee comprised of staff and residents. ADL assistants are considered to be employees of the center, not of its residents. Except for Het Dorp, ADL staff live apart from the residential facility.

One of the curiosities of ADL assistance in Holland's residential center system is the fact that ADL assistants limit their assistance to personal care activities and do not provide assistance with other in-home needs such as laundry and house cleaning. In larger residential centers, this type of assistance may be provided by a housekeeping staff who function very much like hotel maids. In smaller residential centers, this type of assistance must usually be obtained from a community-based home care agency (to be described later).

Meals. Although small meals can be prepared in a person's own dwelling, most meals are arranged on a communal basis. Both large and small residential centers have dining areas with scheduled meal times. ADL assistance is available for those who require assistance with eating.

Required activities (the day activity center). An oddity of Holland's residential center model is the requirement that all residents participate during the day in an outside work, educational, or recreational activity. Very few residents are gainfully employed; some participate in sheltered workshops; most are expected to participate in what is called a "day activity center," usually located a short distance (several kilometers) from the residential center.[3] The typical pattern in the Netherlands is to have a day activity center paired with each residential center. (This pairing of residential and day activity centers is noted by the pairs of dots on the map in Figure 4-1.) Residents are transported by van each morning and returned in the latter part of the afternoon. Transportation is a major cost in operating the residential and day activity center system.

Persons in a day activity center can participate in any one of several dozen activities—crafts, wood working, metal working, publishing a community newsletter, organizing a toy library for the community, listening to records, photography, etc. Most activities appear to be fairly low level, if not insulting to many participants.

The low level of many activities reflects the fact that the day activity cen-

---

3. *Persons unable to produce at least 30% of the production level expected in a sheltered workshop are expected (required) to participate in a day activity center.*

ter concept is a carry over from Holland's huge system of sheltered workshops (80,000 workers) and day activity centers for mentally retarded persons. When the residential center model was implemented with AWBZ financing, many features of the mental retardation service system, also financed by AWBZ, were carried over with little question.

The day activity center system appears demeaning. The implicit assumption is that "busy hands are happy hands" and that residents should, for their own good, get out during the day. Making participation in a day activity center a requirement implies yet another assumption, namely, that disabled persons are not capable of managing their own time and their own affairs. As a result, many residents object to the day activity center requirement; some simply refuse to participate as a matter of principle.

Privacy and sexuality. While the day activity center system appears to be quite backward, other aspects of the residential center model are quite progressive especially in the areas of privacy and human sexuality, both of which are so central to individual personhood.

The respect for privacy begins with each individual being offered their own dwelling and living space with its own street address. As mentioned earlier, neither staff nor ADL assistants can enter any dwelling unless requested or authorized by the resident.

Despite its quasi-institutional character, the residential center model appears to place a high value on human sexuality and recognizes that disabled persons often encounter physical and social barriers in this important area of their lives. Residents who have a sexual partner may require assistance from an ADL worker in preparing for sex, in positioning, or in other special needs. ADL workers are not required to participate in any way that might violate their own value system. Usually a resident will seek out an ADL assistant with whom he or she feels comfortable and feels secure that his or her privacy will be respected.

Persons who do not have a sexual partner, but wish to become more adept and advanced in understanding their own sexuality, can, in some instances secure the services of a surrogate partner usually from an organization or foundation specializing in human sexuality. At one large residential center, for example, a surrogate partner can be obtained at a cost of about f150 ($60) for a 2-hour session. Some centers are more open than others about the use of surrogates, but the prevailing view is that residents are independent people capable of making their own decisions about their own sexuality and that the decisions that residents make in no way reflect the policies of the residential center.

Financing. The average cost for a person to live in a residential center is about f200 ($80) per day for a large center and about f150 ($60) per day for a small center. The average cost for a person to participate in a day activity center is about f125 ($50) per day but is higher in those day activity centers where specialized professional services such as physical therapy are also

Figure 4-1

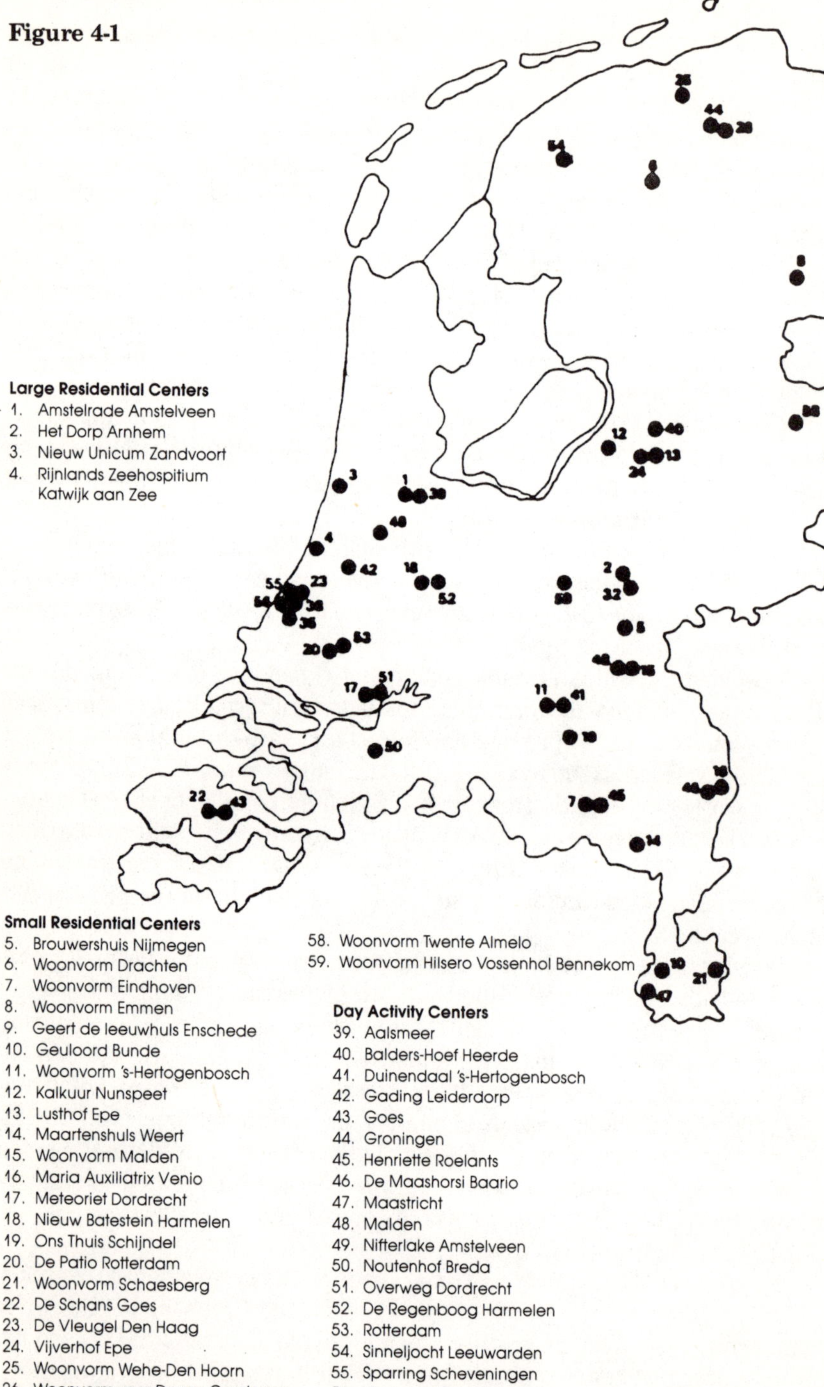

Small Residential Centers

5. Brouwershuis Nijmegen
6. Woonvorm Drachten
7. Woonvorm Eindhoven
8. Woonvorm Emmen
9. Geert de leeuwhuls Enschede
10. Geuloord Bunde
11. Woonvorm 's-Hertogenbosch
12. Kalkuur Nunspeet
13. Lusthof Epe
14. Maartenshuls Weert
15. Woonvorm Malden
16. Maria Auxiliatrix Venio
17. Meteoriet Dordrecht
18. Nieuw Batestein Harmelen
19. Ons Thuis Schijndel
20. De Patio Rotterdam
21. Woonvorm Schaesberg
22. De Schans Goes
23. De Vleugel Den Haag
24. Vijverhof Epe
25. Woonvorm Wehe-Den Hoorn
26. Woonvorm voor Dovan Groningen

58. Woonvorm Twente Almelo
59. Woonvorm Hilsero Vossenhol Bennekom

Day Activity Centers

39. Aalsmeer
40. Balders-Hoef Heerde
41. Duinendaal 's-Hertogenbosch
42. Gading Leiderdorp
43. Goes
44. Groningen
45. Henriette Roelants
46. De Maashorsi Baario
47. Maastricht
48. Malden
49. Nifterlake Amstelveen
50. Noutenhof Breda
51. Overweg Dordrecht
52. De Regenboog Harmelen
53. Rotterdam
54. Sinneljocht Leeuwarden
55. Sparring Scheveningen
56. Vuurvogel Den Haag

available. The bulk of these costs are paid by the AWBZ, Holland's long-term care funding program.[4]

However, each resident is expected to make an offsetting copayment or contribution from his/her WAO or AAW income. This copayment, known as an *eigen bijdrage,* has become quite controversial over the past year or so. Originally the copayment requirement was set low enough (a maximum of f700 or $280 per month) to allow residents discretionary income or ''pocket money'' *(zakgeld)* with which to buy personal care products, to participate in social activities in the community, and to entertain family and friends in their own residences.[5] Because of funding cutbacks and certain abuses,[6] the copayment requirement was raised to f2700 ($1080) per month leaving little or no discretionary income. The decision provoked a huge protest on the part of both residents and residential center operators. As a result, the copayment requirement was later lowered to f1350 ($540) per month, although the issue remains largely unresolved as of this writing. The current copayment requirement allows an individual who only receives AAW benefits to retain about f300 ($120) per month for pocket money.

The upshot of the whole controversy is that the increased copayment requirement is creating a powerful economic incentive for residents to choose less structured living arrangements and thus, also threatens the future viability of the whole residential center system. Accordingly, the final outcome of the copayment controversy is likely to have a major impact on the whole system of residential and IL options available to persons with disabilities.

The Federation

Although independent of one another, the various residential and day activity centers have their own national umbrella organization known as the Dutch Federation of Service Centers for the Physically Handicapped *(Ne-*

---

4. *For a description of the AWBZ, see section III.*

5. *In-home entertainment for family and friends is a very important part of Dutch life. An evening visit, for example, is centered around the consumption of coffee and gebak (a Dutch pastry served when there is sufficient advance notice) often followed by a variety of drinks including a jenever, Holland's very own gin. Moreover, birthdays, another source of in-home entertainment, are required family affairs to which the individual is expected to contribute in one fashion or another. Not to have the financial resources with which to entertain people in one's own home is to diminish one's sense of autonomy and ability to contribute to family and community life.*

6. *The copayment mechanism led to some abuses in the case of mentally retarded persons whose residential care is also paid by the AWBZ. In some instances, mentally retarded persons simply did not spend their discretionary income and eventually amassed significant savings that became a part of an estate assumed by their families upon their death. It is not known how widespread this phenomenon was, but it caused a sense of scandal. In the search for additional funding, the situation prompted policy makers to increase the copayment requirement.*

derlandse Federatie van Voorzieningscentra voor Lichamelijk Gehandi-capten). The Federation provides technical assistance to residential and day activity centers, fosters the development of new centers, and speaks on behalf of its membership before various ministries, councils, and other organizations. In this last capacity, the Federation works closely with the Ministry of Welfare, Public Health, and Culture which supervises the residential and day activity center system.[7]

THE CLUSTERED HOUSING MODEL (FOKUS PROJECTS)

The most prominent force in Holland's system of independent living today is the Fokus Foundation which is responsible for the development of clustered housing projects throughout the Netherlands. Fokus has been very successful in acquiring the political support—both in Parliament and in the various ministries—needed to implement its ideas. The success of Fokus has also had a destabilizing influence on the residential center system and promises to alter IL policy in the Netherlands for years to come.

The Fokus Concept

A single Fokus project consists of 12 to 15 apartments scattered throughout a newly developed housing subdivision usually on the fringes of an expanding urban area. Each Fokus apartment is indistinguishable from other dwelling units within the subdivision except for some of the adaptations made inside the apartment. Because the Netherlands has emphasized neighborhood-based shopping centers in its land use planning, every Fokus dwelling is within easy wheeling distance of a fully accessible shopping center.

Fokus residents are fully integrated into their respective communities. The only feature that sets Fokus residents apart from their neighbors is their link to a "central ADL unit" staffed by ADL assistants. However, this link is reasonably well obscured since the ADL unit, from outside, blends well with its surroundings.

Unlike residents in residential centers, residents in Fokus projects prepare their own meals; they do not eat communally. Nor are residents expected to participate in a day activity center or other program. Fokus residents live independently of one another except for their common link to the central ADL unit.

Origins and Development

The Fokus concept is an import from Sweden where Fokus has flour-

---

7. *The Federation also has regular contact with (1) the Health Insurance Council* (Zieken-fondsraad) *which provides policy direction for the AWBZ program and is the forum in which the copayment requirement is being debated; (2) the Central Hospital Rate Setting Organization* (Centraal Orgaan Ziekenhuistarieven) *which establishes the various per diem rates charged by individual centers; and (3), the NVR, the Dutch Rehabilitation Association (introduced in Section II), of which the Federation is a member organization.*

48

ished for some time. Fokus-Nederland, as it is formally known in the Netherlands, had several false starts as an independent foundation going back to the mid 1970's. Its first project in Almere Haven, an all-new modern city a bit north of Amsterdam, became fully operational in 1980. Each succeeding project has improved on its predecessors in layout, design, and administration.[8] Much of Fokus's early success in the Netherlands has been attributed to the perseverence of its founder, E. vander Hoorst, who until recently also served as Fokus's executive director.

A couple of official milestones in Fokus's history are worth noting:

First was the government's committment in 1980 to support 35 Fokus projects throughout the Netherlands. While the number 35 was a bit artificial, it is now widely accepted as the target number for the next few years. As of early 1984, some of these planned projects were fully operational (see Figure 4-2). To a large extent, the Dutch have gone further than their Swedish counterparts in implementing the Fokus concept, both in number and in character.

Second was the *Clusternota*, a formal document issued by the Ministry of Housing and Land Use Planning in 1981. The *Clusternota* essentially formalized the Fokus model and provided the government's stamp of approval needed for third party funding. More than anything, the *Clusternota* helped to legitimize the Fokus concept in the Netherlands.[9]

Governance

Unlike residential centers, Fokus projects are administered by a single organization. As noted earlier, residential centers are governed by locally established foundations that are federated into a national umbrella group.[10]

The central office staff, located in the northern province of Groningen, is comprised of about a dozen people who are responsible for planning new sites, working with various ministeries, supervising ongoing projects, and publishing a significant bimonthly magazine on disability issues. Once established, local projects work somewhat autonomously with respect to the hiring and supervision of ADL assistants. There is no onsite director. However, the central office does take responsibility for bookkeeping chores (e.g., pay-

---

8. *For example, in some of the earliest projects, all the Fokus apartments are located next to one another; in later projects, they are scattered throughout the subdivision.*

9. *A nota is a government document, usually drafted and sponsored by a lead ministry in consultation with interested parties and becomes the intended policy of government unless disapproved by Parliament. When completed, a nota is published, sometimes in the Staatscourant, a publication much like the Federal Register in the United States.*

10. *Fokus is actually comprised of 3 foundations governing 3 diverse sets of activities: (1) Fokus-Nederland, the parent foundation which establishes and supervises clustered housing projects in keeping with the consumer philosophy; (2) Fokus-Exploitation which provides financial administration for the Fokus system; and (3) Fokus-Consumer Aids which works with suppliers to develop and produce specially adapted equipment and furnishings for Fokus units.*

Figure 4-2

STATUS OF PROJECTS FEBRUARY 1984 CLUSTER PROJECTS

Almere-Haven .... Occupied
Alkmaar
Emmeloord
Nijmegen
Oss
Groningen-Beyum — 14 projects occupied
Purmerend
Utrecht I
Zoetermeer
Almere-Stad I
Rotterdam
Groningen-Paddepoel
Nieuwegein
Doetinchem

Construction phase ....
Drachten
Tilburg
Amersfoort
Amsterdam I
Amsterdam II
Venlo
Dordrecht

Ready for construction...........
Lelystad
Roosendaal
Den Bosch

Planning phase.................
Amstelveen
Middelburg
Kerkrade
Arnhem
Eindhoven
Zwolle
Enschede
Utrecht II
Almere-Stad II

Initiative phase.................
Den Haag
Goes
35 projects in total

roll, social insurance premiums, vacation time, and billings). According to Fokus management philosophy, the central office also serves as the guardian of the "Fokus concept." This guardianship role was designed, in part, to prevent what had happened in Sweden where autonomous local projects sometimes degenerated into mini institutions with ADL staff beginning to take on the characteristics of a medical team with "team meetings" to discuss the well-being of each resident. Learning from the Swedish experience, Fokus-Nederland has attempted to prevent its ADL staffs from lapsing into the medical model as well-intentioned people sometimes do.

There are no residents councils. The ongoing relationship between Fokus and its residents is more akin to a landlord-tenant relationship with the added services of ADL assistants.

Eligibility Criteria

There are two main eligibility criteria. First, a person must be between 18 and 65 years old to move into a Fokus apartment. The age criterion is a function of the fact that ADL assistance is paid by the AAW program which is targeted to working age persons. However, persons who become 65 years while a resident can remain a resident. Second, a person must require at least 10, but not more than 30 hours, of ADL assistance per week. In practice, this criterion is sometimes waived but a limitation in self-care remains central to defining who can live in Fokus.

There are no other formal criteria. Even prolonged institutionalization, with all its adverse effects, is not cause for denial. It is generally assumed that if a person has gone through the trouble of submitting an application and a personal interview—knowing that he/she will have to arrange his/her own meals, food shopping, and other home maintenance chores, he/she also possesses the motivation to get out of an institution and should not be denied the opportunity to do so. The Fokus philosophy is that each individual should be given the chance to succeed, and for that matter, to fail.

ADL Assistance

The model of ADL assistance used in the Fokus system is essentially the same as the model used in the residential center system, i.e., the use of centralized, 24-hour, on-call ADL assistants. The central ADL unit is usually staffed at all times by at least 2 persons working in slightly overlapping shifts. An ADL assistant can be summoned by the resident with the use of a push button, telephone-like device that signals the central ADL unit to indicate who is calling. ADL assistants also carry a communication device that allows them to communicate with residents when they are away from the central ADL unit. If an ADL assistant is not immediately available, the resident can be advised as to how soon an ADL assistant will be coming along.

ADL assistants, like their counterparts in the residential center system, are paid the minimum wage with some adjustment for evening and weekend work. Most are younger or middle working age women.[11] ADL assistants receive no special training on the assumption that their tasks are everyday tasks already learned in early childhood, and on the assumption that individual residents are perfectly capable of directing their own care. From casual conversation, it appears that ADL assistants are very much committed to the concept of self-direction and share the residents views on their right to live independently.

An interesting aspect of the Fokus model is the physical layout of the central ADL unit. Aside from the "office area" from which ADL assistants work, there is a kitchen area, a dining and meeting area, a laundry room, a bathroom, and bathing room.[12] Most of these facilities duplicate, to some degree, what is already available in the resident's own home. The dining and meeting area, according to one observer, is a carryover from the Swedish version of Fokus, and appears to be based on the assumption that residents wish to meet as a group and have a group identity around which to socialize. However, just the opposite has occurred. Residents seldom socialize as a group and in many instances barely know one another. Moreover, the availability of a central dining and meeting area appears to run counter to the Dutch tradition of entertaining in one's own home. In some Fokus projects, one can find the dining area closet loaded with dinnerware that has never been used. It appears that Fokus has been sufficiently successful at social integration that it might do well to reconsider some of the physical features of the central ADL unit carried over from the Swedish version.

Financing

Like his/her able-bodied neighbors, each Fokus resident leases his/her apartment through a housing rental corporation known as a *woningbouwvereniging*. Monthly rent can amount to as much as f750 ($300) per month, still quite modest given the spaciousness of most Fokus apartments. In addition, each resident is responsible for paying his/her own utilities (about f250 or $100 per month) and telephone. For most individuals, these costs must be paid from their WAO or AAW income. Individuals, whose incomes are too low relative to their housing costs, can obtain a rent subsidy.

---

11. Dutch women participate in the labor force to a much lesser degree than women in other western industrialized countries. When they do participate, they participate mainly to supplement family income. They seldom view their income as an important source of income, a view also reflected in Dutch tax and social policy which has traditionally treated women-earned second incomes more harshly than men-earned first incomes. Despite their concern for equity in most areas of social policy, the Dutch, by American standards, have not been very "progressive" when it comes to women issues. This arises, in part, because, in measuring social equity, the family or household, rather than the individual, is usually the unit of observation.

12. The central feature of the bathing room is an oversized bathtub into which a person can be lowered with the use of a hydraulic chair.

The structure known as central ADL unit is subsidized by the Ministry of Housing, Land Use Planning, and Environmental Policy and is leased by Fokus from the housing rental corporation for a nominal sum of 1 guilder per year.

ADL assistance is financed as an in-kind benefit through the AAW. While the resident is viewed as the AAW beneficiary, the actual payment is made to Fokus as the employing organization. Fokus, through its central office, maintains a computerized system which tracks each ADL assistant's hours and work history for the purpose of complying with Holland's complicated labor laws with respect to the computation of vacation time, vacation allowances, social insurance premiums, and income taxes. The cost of ADL assistance, for billing purposes, is f28 ($11) per hour. This figure includes wages, fringe benefits, and other costs including a portion of Fokus's central office operation involved in supervising the ADL assistance program.

Paying for ADL assistance through the AAW represents a significant departure from the usual method of financing such services through the AWBZ as in the residential center model. AAW financing has important symbolic value as well. It serves notice that ADL assistance should not be viewed as an extension of the medical care delivery system as is implied by the AWBZ program. Moreover, AAW financing frees residents from AWBZ-required out-of-home activities noted in our discussion regarding the residential center model.

Unfortunately, AAW-financed ADL assistance cannot be obtained outside of a clustered housing project, i.e., Fokus. Individuals living on their own, apart from a Fokus project, must obtain their ADL assistance from friends and relatives or, if lucky, from a community-based home help agency. The alternatives available to these individuals will be explored in the discussion on the independent housing model which follows.

THE INDEPENDENT HOUSING MODEL

In the absence of hard statistics, it is difficult to determine how many persons needing daily ADL assistance are living on their own apart from an organized housing program. The prevailing view is that the number of such individuals is quite small although there are some who believe the number to be quite large. Regardless of their number, persons living independently of an organized program are usually left to their own wits as to how their ADL assistance will be provided: most rely on a spouse, a friend, a neighbor, or another family member, and seek supplementary assistance from a home help agency when the main ADL provider is ill or away from home.

Interestingly, a person living in this fashion can usually acquire funding for home modifications and adapted private transportation but not for ADL assistance, a state of affairs that will be addressed in the last section of this monograph.

The Netherlands has one of the most extensive systems of home help agencies in the world that routinely provides an array of in-home services such as infant care on behalf of new mothers *(kraamzorg)*, child care on behalf of a hospitalized parent, personal care for a recently hospitalized adult, care for an older person trying to delay institutionalization, and others. Yet, this system has failed to reach the ongoing needs of persons requiring routine ADL assistance. My purpose here is to consider the scope of the home help system and to evaluate its residual capacities to address the in-home needs of nonelderly persons with severe self-care limitations.

As in the United States, the home help system is comprised of two main types of organizations: (1) home health *(gezondeidszorg)* agencies and (2) home care *(gezinsverzorging)* agencies comparable to homemaker/chore service agencies in the United States. The distinction in the kinds of services rendered by these two types of organizations is sometimes a bit artificial and is, as in the United States, a source of fierce professional and territorial disputes that have also compromised the ability of home help agencies to be more responsive to the in-home needs of persons with severe physical disabilities.

Home Health Services *(Kruiswerk)*

Home health care is an integral part of Holland's primary health care system *(eerstelijnszorg)*. Home health services are organized by district following the neighborhood boundaries or districts into which many Dutch towns are divided.[13] Holland's 4000 district nurses *(wijkverpleegsters)*—about 1 nurse per 3500 population—are the backbone of home health system. District nurses work closely with local primary care physicians or "house doctors" *(huisartsen)* who literally make house calls.

District nurses are salaried employees of home health agencies known as *kruiswerk organisaties*, literally, "cross work" organizations, a term dating back to the time when home health agencies were organized along strict confessional lines with each confessional group having a different colored cross in its flag following the example of the international Red Cross.[14] Prior to deconfessionalization in the mid 1970's (see section II), all 3 main confessional home health agencies could exist side by side in the same community leading to a tremendous duplication of services. One benefit of deconfessionalization has been the ability to secure greater organizational consolidation and a more efficient delivery of services.

Most home health agencies provide a wide variety of services—routine nursing care, physical therapy referral, ADL assistance, range of motion exercises, injections, and the like. However, most services are directed to con-

---

13. *In addition to district-based staffs, Holland's home health system also has a hierarchy of regional, provincial, and national offices.*

14. *Protestants had an orange and green cross, Catholics had a yellow and white cross, and the unaffiliated had a green cross.*

ditions that tend to be acute or episodic in nature, not to conditions that tend to be chronic and continuing. Long-term cases are discouraged and services are usually only provided between 8 am and 6 pm each day. Some home health agencies are beginning to experiment with extended hours and on-call services. For the most part, ADL assistance from home health agencies is not routinely available to persons with severe disabilities except in a very supplementary, *ad hoc,* fashion. Home health agencies see long-term ADL assistance as a drain on their resources that diminishes their capacity to reach a wider segment of the population.

Each direct service worker, i.e. district nurse, costs approximately f50 ($20) per hour or about f100.000 ($40,000) per year after social insurance premiums and agency overhead costs are taken into account. About 2/3 of these costs are paid by the AWBZ. The other 1/3 of these costs are paid from annual membership dues of about f40 ($16) per family. Most Dutch families are members, a habit that dates back to the time when people participated because of confessional loyalties. Member families receive home health services without charge. However, home health care is slowly moving from the voluntary sector to the public sector as older confessional loyalties diminish and as public financing takes up a larger share of each agency's budget.

Yet, their reliance on membership dues indicates that home health agencies are still broad-based. Unfortunately, a broad-based, dues-paying constituency also means that, when it comes to allocating their limited resources, home health agencies will have every incentive, politically and financially, to meet the few needs of many, and not the many needs of a few such as persons with life-long disabilities.

Home Care Services *(Gezinsverzorging)*[15]

Home care services are organized much like home health services with district, regional, provincial, and national offices. Like home health agencies, home care agencies were originally organized along confessional lines which led to a tremendous proliferation of agencies during the post-war period. However, as noted in Section II, deconfessionalization has led to considerable consolidation: from more than 900 agencies prior to 1970 to 241 in 1983.

Home care services are provided mainly by 2 types of direct service providers, homemakers and chore service workers. Homemakers are agency employees especially trained to work with selected client groups such as older persons and families without mothers. Chore service workers, known as *alpha helpsters,* are hired directly by the client to do ordinary household chores—general house cleaning, food shopping, some meal preparation, laundry, and other light chores. The role of the agency is to evaluate the client's need for chore services and to help recruit a chore service worker. In a

---

15. *A more literal translation of the term* ''Gezinsverzorging'' *would be* ''*family care.*''

sense, the agency serves as a broker in the chore service market trying to bring the demand (need) and supply sides of the market together. In the case where the home care agency is unable to recruit a chore service worker, the disabled person is free to obtain his/her own source of chore services after income eligibility is determined and a needs assessment is completed. Unlike homemakers, chore service workers receive no special training. From the standpoint of disabled persons living independently, chore service workers are the more important source of in-home assistance.

Homemakers and chore service workers also provide in-home assistance to persons with disabilities such as those living in a residential center or Fokus project. As mentioned earlier, non-ADL forms of assistance must be obtained from an outside source. Each individual is expected to arrange his/her own source of non-ADL assistance which, in most cases, is a chore service worker from a home care agency.

For persons living in independent housing apart from a residential center or Fokus project, chore service workers will provide limited ADL assistance but only as an extension of their other tasks. However, chore service workers do not provide ADL assistance routinely since to do so treads on the turf usually reserved for home health agencies.

As in the case of home health services, home care services are usually limited to working hours, 8 am to 6 pm. However, in situations where disabled persons recruit their own chore service worker, there is no restriction as to hours of assistance.

The AAW will pay for chore services for those persons who are AAW eligible, which includes most disabled persons 65 years and under. For others, payment requirements are scaled according to income with different scales for single individuals and families. The maximum charge is about f9,50 ($3.80) per hour; actual costs are about f30 ($12) per hour when agency costs are factored in. However, in the case where a person recruits his or her chore service worker, actual costs are closer to f15 ($6) per hour. There is no upper income limit in determining eligibility; the service is universally available.

Reaching the Person with a Severe Disability

For the most part, Holland's home help industry—both home health and home care agencies—has not viewed the severely disabled person requiring help with personal care as a target client group. These individuals require sustained, uninterrupted, and integrated daily assistance which is not in keeping with the more intermittent, episodic model of care assumed by most agencies. The question remains as to what potential there may exist within the home help system to meet both the personal care and housekeeping needs of persons with self-care limitations in a sustained and integrated fashion. A few barriers are worth noting:

First, the line between ADL assistance and housekeeping is sharply drawn for professional and financial reasons. Home health nurses, for example, see themselves as professionally trained persons qualified to provide hands on care. The use of "untrained" and "unqualified" personnel, such as chore service workers, to provide similar care violates a sense of professional turf. The distinction between ADL assistance and other forms of in-home assistance is reinforced by the dual funding system in which AWBZ pays for home health services and the AAW pays for housekeeping types of tasks.

Second, both home health and home care agencies have limited hours of service, usually 8 to 6, which does not correspond to the lifestyle and needs of most persons with disabilities, especially those who are vocationally active and must be at their place of employment during regular working hours. Unfortunately, there are severe economic disincentives to extending the hours of coverage beyond the 8-to-6 working day: evening shifts must be paid 125% of the usual hourly rate; the night shift 150%, and weekend shifts 200%. Moreover, most home help services are provided by women who, in Dutch society, have more well-defined family routines during early and mid evening hours than their American counterparts.

Third, Holland's home help industry has embraced the concepts of *zelfzorg* (self-care) and *mantelzorg* (environmental care).[16] Both concepts attempt to put more of the burden of home help back on the individual and his/her environmental support system, i.e., family, neighbors, and friends. Agency organized home help services are viewed as supplementary to the services provided by a person's social support system. When applying for home help services, a person's social support system is carefully evaluated. The consideration of a person's social support system is, in part, precipitated by funding cutbacks and has been a convenient way of stretching limited funds. However, the concepts of *zelfzorg* and *mantelzorg* are not always appropriate to disabled persons requiring daily ADL assistance. In fact, the goal of home help services for such individuals is to enable individuals to become more independent of family supports, especially for young adults who need to establish their own households and a lifestyle that is independent of parental control. All too often *mantelzorg*, or more specifically, family care, merely perpetuates the parent-child relationship into adulthood and may even precipitate unnecessary institutionalization when an aging parental caregiver is no longer able to provide the care he or she once did.[17]

One attempt to get beyond some of these barriers is the 3 pilot projects undertaken by what is now the Ministry of Welfare, Public Health, & Culture and the home care agencies in 3 cities—Delft, Enschede, and Groningen. One purpose of the projects was to determine if the home care system could be ex-

---

16. Mantel *literally means "coat" and refers to the social and environmental support system in which a person is "wrapped."*

17. *An analogous situation may occur in the case of a person dependent on his or her spouse for ADL assistance. In such cases, the day-to-day demands of such care can result in unnecessary stresses leading to the dissolution of the marriage relationship.*

panded in two main directions: (1) to extend the hours of service beyond the traditional working hours of 8 to 6; and (2) to include both ADL assistance and housekeeping tasks. However, the projects are basically "cluster projects" since each serves a cluster of about 6 disabled persons living in a newly built housing development. In a sense, they are much like Fokus projects except that the in-home assistance is provided by a local home care agency instead of Fokus employees. The projects began in 1975 as demonstration projects and were evaluated in 1978 but have since not been expanded since Fokus has been given, more or less, the exclusive right to provide ADL assistance on a cluster basis. So as not to jeopardize the well-being of those who were in the original pilot projects, the Ministry continues to fund each of the original 3 projects with special grants.[18]

Although 24-hour coverage is provided in each project there still is not the full integration of ADL and housekeeping tasks. In the Enschede project, for example, the local home health agency provides ADL assistance during the morning hours and the local home care agency provides ADL assistance during the balance of the day in conjunction with other housekeeping tasks.

The 3 projects represent an honest attempt on the part of home help agencies to meet the needs of disabled persons requiring ongoing in-home assistance. However, Holland's home help system has not been fully responsive to the ongoing in-home needs of those seeking to live independently of a cluster project. The failure to be more responsive not only reflects important policy differences among provider agencies and funding sources but also very human factors including professional status, territoriality, and simple oversight because of training or background. Yet, in all fairness, it should be mentioned that Holland's home help system is, in some instances, beginning to provide more integrated in-home care and more flexible hours of service.

In the next and final section of the monograph we will consider some of the options available to Holland's home help system in the context of Holland's overall 3-part residential and IL system and in the light of prevailing attempts to cutback the scope of Holland's public sector. These considerations will also lay the foundation for evaluating the short- and long-term implications for the United States.

----

18. *In a sense the 3 projects could be viewed as a 4th model in Holland's residential and IL system, albeit a hybrid one that takes elements from the cluster model and the independent housing model. Because the 3 projects are not national in scope, they were not given separate consideration for purposes of this monograph.*

V THE FUTURE OF DUTCH IL POLICY & ITS IMPLICATIONS FOR THE UNITED STATES

The Netherlands appears uncertain about the future of its policies toward persons with disabilites. Much of existing policy is based on a willingness of the general population to extend the benefits of postwar prosperity to more vulnerable groups in society. This willingness was based on a sense of moral commitment—often religious in origin—and on a sense of certainty that the economic prosperity would continue indefinitely. The depth of the present recession has eroded that sense of certainty. Moreover, unlike years past, there appears to be little in the Dutch economy that will give it the cutting edge it needs to excel in world markets so essential to an economy dependent on world trade. The present uncertainty has contributed to a greater willingness to question the scope of existing cash and in-kind programs directed to disabled persons.

Yet, these programs are part of a larger "safety net" in which all persons participate and in which all persons have a stake. High unemployment and tight labor markets, for even the best trained in Holland's labor force, have contributed to a sense of mutual economic vulnerability and, perhaps, to a mutual hesitancy to drastically change the overall structure of Holland's social welfare system. Thus, the probable impact of current economic conditions and public opinion upon Holland's residential care and IL system for disabled persons is hard to predict.

While the future impact of these exogeneous variables is difficult to evaluate, there are several more endogenous variables, e.g., reimbursement policies, that are more likely to have an impact on Holland's residential and IL system in the foreseeable future. The probable impact of these endogenous variables also has much to suggest as to what the implications of Holland's residential and IL system might be for a country such as the United States. Accordingly, the purpose of this section is to (1) consider the future of Holland's residential and IL system and (2) ascertain the implications of the system for the United States.

THE FUTURE OF INDEPENDENT LIVING IN THE NETHERLANDS

The future of independent living in the Netherlands is best understood by considering each of Holland's residential and IL models as part of a larger system of competing models. The relative advantages and disadvantages that each model brings to this competition provide important clues about the future of independent living in the Netherlands. Presently, most "market conditions" favor less restrictive and more independent alternatives.

Future of the Residential Center Model

The residential center model is under tremendous pressure from at least 3 sources. First, many persons with disabilities, over the years, are simply prefering less restrictive, less stigmatizing, and more independent lifestyles. Requirements such as participation in a day activity center are viewed as infringements on personal autonomy and inconsistent with the IL aspirations of persons with disabilities. Second, the increase in copayment requirements *(eigen bijdrage)* under the AWBZ program creates powerful economic incentives for residents to seek alternatives to the residential center model. Third, the Fokus system, with its roomy apartments, provides a more atractive and more independent alternative for residents of existing residential centers.

Under present conditions it is doubtful that a large center such as Het Dorp will survive in its present form or whether it can survive at all. Competition from smaller residential centers and Fokus projects has already resulted in excess capacity—some estimate that as many as 60 of the 450 units are now vacant.

Even smaller centers will begin to feel such pressure and may soon experience excess capacity. Attempts to shore up the residential center model with formalized functional and developmental concepts—as was recently done to enhance the model's credibility and legitimacy (WVC: 1983)—will not stem the tide. The future of residential centers may be one of transitional facilities for persons in various stages of transition as in the case of young adults in transition from living with protective parents to living independently. Still, residential centers are being built when future market conditions would indicate otherwise.

For the foreseeable future, most of the pressure on the residential model will be coming from the Fokus system. With only 14 operational projects (approximately 200 residents), the Fokus system has already provoked considerable anxiety within the residential center system. One is only left to speculate as to what kind of pressure will be exerted on the system when all 35 proposed projects (approximately 500 residents) become operational. According to Fokus officials there are some 1,200 persons on Fokus's waiting list. Many of these persons are reported to be currently living in residential centers.

The Future of the Fokus Model

The Fokus model is clearly in the ascendancy at this moment. Its apartments are attractive and it provides a secure source of ADL assistance. More importantly, the Fokus Foundation has effectively made the Fokus model synonomous with independent living. Fokus has been a leader in advocating for the IL aspirations of disabled persons and has effectively used its bimonthly publication, *Brandpunt*, in doing so. Also, Fokus is politically well connected and has enjoyed the confidence of cooperating ministries.

Fokus has, from time to time, come under criticism. The criticism has come mainly from two sources. The first source, in the early stage of Fokus's development in the Netherlands, came from those who questioned the ability of disabled persons to live independently without supervision. By fighting this issue, Fokus quickly became the champion of self-determination. The second source of criticism comes from those who criticize Fokus as an organization—for its various conflicts of interest or the manner in which it works with local groups. It is beyond the scope of this monograph to address these criticisms except to say that they arise, in part, from a highly competitive, highly charged atmosphere and clearly illustrate the tenseness within the overall residential and IL system.

Fokus has been very successful and deserves credit for advancing the range of alternatives to persons with disabilities in the Netherlands. However, one does wonder if the Fokus model has not been implemented too rigidly. Although there is some variation as to how project sites are layed out, each project site is virtually a carbon copy of the other with respect to its ADL assistance program. To illustrate, each ADL staff maintains an identical working schedule. Thus, it is possible that certain persons will not be accepted into a project if their ADL needs do not coincide with the residual capacities of the central ADL unit. The similarity of project-to-project working schedules may be important from the standpoint of a system that is centrally supervised from a remote location but may not always be in keeping with the needs of potential residents. Certainly, some degree of economy can be obtained with standardization. Nonetheless, as Fokus continues to grow, it may have to regionalize the administration of its projects, an outcome that may contribute to greater flexibility at the local level.

In many respects, Fokus is now viewed, in some quarters, as "the solution." The tendency in the Netherlands has been to seize upon a single model as the final solution. This was Holland's fatal flaw when it began Het Dorp more than 2 decades ago. The lesson of Het Dorp is that the Netherlands would do well in viewing the Fokus model as an important step in expanding IL alternatives for persons with disabilities.

The Future of Independent Housing

The future of independent housing will depend largely on whether in-home attendant care will become routinely available outside a residential center or cluster project. There are 2 potential suppliers of in-home attendant care: (1) the existing home help system and (2) some other source yet to be determined.

The future capacity of Holland's home help system is somewhat doubtful unless the system can overcome some of the barriers mentioned in Section IV: (1) the sharp line drawn between ADL and other forms of assistance; (2) the limited hours of service, from 8 a.m. to 6 p.m.; and (3) the renewed emphasis on the use of family and environmental supports which may not be appropriate for disabled persons seeking to become more independent from family and neighborhood charity.

However, the main barrier to meeting the in-home needs of disabled persons living on their own is Holland's overwhelming fixation on just one model of in-home assistance, namely, the model of central ADL assistance. It is a model of care that cuts across all 3 major living alternatives now available to disabled persons in the Netherlands—in residential centers, in Fokus projects, and even in the 3 demonstration projects administered in conjunction with home help agencies.

The Netherlands has yet to seriously consider alternative models of in-home assistance such as the one-on-one attendant care model where persons are paid to obtain and manage their own ADL assistants (usually more than one with some serving as ''back-ups'') subject to need criteria based on functional capacity. This mode of assistance has become increasingly popular in the United States over the last several years as the IL movement has gained strength. The features of the one-on-one model can perhaps be best understood when contrasted with the central ADL model as in Figure 5-1.

In the central ADL model, the ADL assistant is first and foremost an employee of the foundation or *stichting* which hires, fires, and supervises the ADL assistant. However, the ADL assistant works at the direction of *both* the *stichting* and the resident. In the central ADL model, assistance is viewed more as an extended medical benefit when financed by the AWBZ program (as in residential centers) and more as a social benefit when financed by the AAW program (as in Fokus projects). Except in the 3 demonstration projects, ADL assistants are limited to providing only personal care services—bathing, grooming, dressing, etc., not other forms of in-home assistance.

In the one-on-one attendant model, the attendant is a self-employed individual hired, fired, and supervised by the disabled person. The attendant works solely at the direction of the disabled person. The service is viewed as a social benefit. Attendants are not limited to providing personal care but also various chore services depending on the person's family circumstances.

Although the one-on-one attendant care model has rapidly become the preferred model of assistance among disabled persons in the United States, this observer found the model to simply be beyond the comprehension of many in the Netherlands. When probing to find out why, this observer uncovered a deep-down, sometimes unspoken, mistrust of disabled persons to fully direct and manage their own affairs. By the same token, Americans have overlooked some merits of the central ADL model, a matter to be taken up when the implications for the United States are discussed.

If a one-on-one model were implemented in the Netherlands, the determination of need—usually expressed in hours per day or per week—could be the responsibility of the GMD (Joint Medical Service) and delegated to a home help agency or to a Fokus-type organization. Need could be reevaluated once a year unless circumstances required otherwise.

An embryonic version of the one-on-one attendant model already exists in the Netherlands in the form of *alpha helpsters* or chore service workers who are paid by home care agencies but employed by care receivers (see Section IV). By slightly altering the conditions of employment and by expanding

Contrasting Models of In-home Assistance
for Disabled Persons

Central ADL Model (Neth.)	**One-on-one Attendant Care (U.S.)**
• Assistant hired & fired by *stichting*	• Attendant hired & fired by disabled person
• Assistant employed & supervised by *stichting*	• Attendant self-employed & supervised by disabled person
• Provision of care directed by both disabled person & *stichting*	• Provision of care directed by disabled person
• Payment for services made to *stichting* which in turn pays assistant	• Payment for services made to disabled person who in turn pays attendant
• Disabled person considered a resident	• Disabled person considered a consumer
• Includes only personal care activities, not housekeeping chores	• Includes both personal care and housekeeping activites
• Viewed as a medical (AWBZ) or social (AAW) benefit	• Viewed as a social benefit

Figure 5-1

chore service work to include personal care, one would in effect establish a bona fide model of one-on-one attendant care as described above.[1]

As noted in Section IV, the Dutch home help system has, in recent years, paid considerable attention to the concept of self-care (*zelf/zorg*). In its more restrictive sense, the concept of self-care refers to the ability of the individual to actually perform various self-care activities, from toileting to dressing. However, the concept of self-care needs to be expanded, if not redefined: Self-care is more than the mere performance of self-care tasks, but rather, the control and direction a person can have in managing his/her own bodily care. Self-care is not mere independence in performing personal care activities, but independence in managing one's own personal care.

In an era of "cutback government," it is increasingly likely that the Netherlands will begin to look at other models of in-home assistance— models that require less day-to-day agency management and that will, accordingly, cost less but will also be in accord with the IL aspirations of the country's most disabled citizens.

IMPLICATIONS FOR THE UNITED STATES

Cultural differences often preclude the simple transplantation of program concepts and models from one country to another. By the same token, cultural differences should not be an excuse to simply dismiss ideas from another country. There are several features of the Dutch system that merit further consideration in the United States: (1) the use of the centralized ADL assistance and clustered housing for selected groups of individuals, (2) the employment status of ADL assistants, (3) the financing of in-kind benefits, (4) the difficulties arising from the provision of residential care services, and (5) the "corporatist system" of decision making in disability policy.

Centralized ADL Assistance & Clustered Housing

We have already noted how the Dutch have overlooked the one-on-one method of attendant care. Yet, with a few exceptions, Americans have overlooked the merits of centralized ADL assistance as provided in the clustered housing model. Centralized ADL assistance and clustered housing deserve further consideration in the United States for at least 2 groups of individuals —and others who, for lifestyle reasons, would prefer a more secure source of attendant care.

The first group is persons needing respirator assistance. For the first

---

1. *Moreover, the Dutch are very much accustomed to arranging their own in-home services on a private basis in the "underground economy" by hiring* werksters *who assist in performing various domestic chores. However, the acquisition of such services are often laced with overt and covert class distinctions that cannot be recommended as a basis for social policy.*

High levels of unemployment, among the highest in Europe, would also suggest a ready supply of persons, especially younger persons, who could be employed by disabled persons to perform in-home tasks.

time since the polio days, the United States is experiencing a burgeoning number of respirator users—among persons with high level spinal cord injury, persons with end-stage muscular dystrophy who choose to continue living, persons with amyolateralsclerosis who also wish to extend their lives, and low birthweight newborns who survive but require permanent respirator assistance. The survival of these groups in recent years reflects changing technologies and the changing values of both disabled persons and medical practitioners.[2]

Post-polio survivors are perhaps the best example we have of how respirator users, over the years, have managed to live independently and arrange the attendant care they need. However, persons without an extended family and social support system often need a more secure source of attendant care than what can ordinarily be rendered in a one-on-one system of attendant care. Many persons using a respirator may only need a limited amount of direct assistance per day—perhaps 4 to 7 hours—but often still need 24-hour back-up for intermittent assistance and in the event their life-support system should malfunction. For such individuals, centralized ADL assistance, provided in a clustered housing setting, should be explored as a serious option.

The second group in the United States is persons who are working. Many working disabled persons prefer to put their energy into their jobs and simply do not want to be bothered having to worry about their day-to-day source of attendant care. Locating a continuous source of attendants and back-ups can be a hassle, especially when an individual feels there are more productive things to do with his or her time.

I am not recommending small ghettos of respirator users or other attendant care consumers. However, I do believe that clustered housing with centralized attendant care should be considered, with some modification, as one of the options available to persons with disabilities.

The Employment Status of Attendants

One troublesome issue in the United States is the employment status of attendants. Most are low-paid, part-time workers. The needs of attendants have not been adequately recognized in the United States. By contrast, ADL assistants in the Netherlands are recognized as bona fide employees entitled to a ''minimum wage''[3] with certain protections and benefits. Although I am not prepared to recommend the more costly Dutch approach, I do believe that the contrast between the Netherlands and the United States highlights the extent to which the needs of attendants have been ignored. Perhaps at-

---

2. *Significant groups of respirator users are not to be found in the Netherlands as they are emerging in the United States.*

3. *The minimum wage in the Netherlands is not to be confused with the minimum wage in the United States. The minimum wage in the Netherlands is more akin to a minimum standard of living on the basis of which income benefits and wage rates are determined.*

tendants in the United States will, and should, come mainly from persons in various stages of transition and willing to work part-time, e.g., college students. Still, a more adequate level of compensation is needed. A more adequate wage rate will also guarantee a more willing and secure supply of attendants for disabled persons. A higher wage rate may reduce the force of the frequently used benefit-cost argument used by many who promote attendant care as an alternative to institutional care. However, the needs of attendants deserve consideration as do the needs of persons with disabilities.

The Financing of In-kind Benefits

One of the features of the Dutch system observed in Section III was the extent to which in-kind benefits (e.g., assistive devices, adapted private transportation) are viewed as entitlements and financed through Holland's entitlement programs. Moreover, it was noted how the Joint Medical Service or GMD serves as a single point of entry for the acquisition of most in-kind benefits so essential to a person's ability to live independently. In the United States, by contrast, in-kind benefits are not viewed as entitlements and must be secured from a variety of sources, often on a means-tested basis.

One of the more important sources of in-kind benefits in the United States is the federal-state vocational rehabilitation system. Despite the miniature Title VII IL program administered under the Rehabilitation Act, state rehabilitation agencies remain first and foremost vocational rehabilitation agencies with fixed budgets that do not dispose agencies to dispense scarce resources essential to independent living. Moreover, there is the ever present tendency to wait and see if some other funding source will pick up the tab.

The Dutch single-entry and single-source funding system for most in-kind benefits deserves full consideration in the United States. More specifically consideration should be given to the following alternatives: (1) expanding state vocational rehabilitation authority to include the routine provision of nonvocationally related in-kind benefits; (2) establishing a funding mechanism as an adjunct to the existing disability income system, i.e., SSDI and SSI; or (3) establishing an entirely separate authority offering one-stop evaluation and financing of all in-kind benefits including durable medical equipment.

The failure to obtain these benefits from a single source has been a major frustration for disabled Americans. Moreover, the present piecemeal approach has been expensive; it precludes a comprehensive review of individual needs in a way that will permit economic trade-offs in choosing, for example, varying amounts of attendant care and home adaptations.

The Dutch experience, however, indicates that a single-source approach can have its difficulties: It gives the evaluation agency a "monopoly" position that can discourage the introduction of new technologies. Suppliers with new products of interest to disabled persons sometimes cannot get their devices on the "approved list."

The Use of Residential Centers

The Dutch experience with residential centers offers an object lesson. The Netherlands has invested heavily in residential centers. Despite some of its redeeming features, the residential center model is now becoming a drag on the whole residential and IL system as persons begin to opt for more independent living arrangements. The lesson is clear: investments in brick and mortar have a way of continuing programs beyond the time they are needed or wanted. They introduce rigidities in the market that later come to be regretted. Residential care is not the way to go.

The Corporatist System of Decision Making

In Section II it was noted how various disability interests—consumers and providers—are organized into umbrella organizations which in turn are represented on various boards, ministerial steering committees, and semi-independent councils. We also noted how the consensus forged in these deliberative bodies is considered sufficiently binding to be ratified by Parliament without much alteration.

Although this system has been criticized for having created an extra-parliamentary form of government, all affected groups are guaranteed at least some degree of representation. The same cannot be said for the United States where provider and consumer interests are represented only to the extent to which they are sufficiently funded or politically connected to make some impact on policy. Too much of the American system of interest group politics is determined by the economic muscle each group brings to the process.

Consumer interests have seldom been well represented in the American political process. Consumer groups such as the American Coalitions of Citizens with Disabilities (ACCD)—the American counterpart to the Dutch Handicapped Council introduced in Section II—have had mixed success in representing consumer interests. ACCD's impact in the policy making process has varied with the economic health of the organization as measured by its funding base and staffing. When consumer organizations begin to lose their funding base, they are perceived as weak and can be more easily passed over in the policy consultation process.

This is less true in the Netherlands where consumer organizations are organized into umbrella groups who act as recognized bargaining agents for their respective member organizations. Consumer organizations are accorded a legitimacy that is not soley dependent on the size of its budget or staff.

Fragments of the corporatist model can be found in the American system in the form of the National Council on the Handicapped which provides policy leadership for the Rehabilitation Services Administration and the National Institute for Handicapped Research. Unlike its closest Dutch counterpart—the Interministerial Steering Committee mentioned in Section II—members of the National Council are symbolic representatives who serve at the pleasure of the President, not by vote of their respective organizations. Consensus and decisions forged within the National Council are in no way binding on the Congress. Moreover, as presidential appointees, members of the National Council are expected to be at least somewhat deferential to the wishes of the Administration in power.

Although representative government, i.e., the U.S. Congress, should not be undermined, the Dutch experience does suggest that strengthening the National Council would be one way in which the interests of disabled persons might be enhanced and protected from the erratic political winds that sometimes blow across the national political landscape. Two suggestions come to mind: (1) the appointment of members representing well-defined consumer and provider interests balanced with persons whose interests are less vested as in the case of ''crown members'' appointed to Dutch consultative councils; (2) the appointment of senators and representatives of sufficiently diverse views such that the consensus forged by the Council would be considered binding on the Congress. Incidently, this was exactly the strategy used by the President when he appointed the Social Security Commission which forged the consensus on long-term funding issues, a consensus ratified by Congress with little debate.

I do not want to suggest such a consultation process in every policy area nor do I want to encourage the proliferation of such consultative bodies as has been the Dutch experience. However, the needs of disabled persons are compelling and deserve special consideration within our system of policy making.

IN CLOSING

Aside from any deficiencies in Holland's residential and IL system, one factor stands out: a remarkable consensus in nearly all sectors in society that persons with severe disabilities should be accorded an adequate standard of living in keeping with the standards enjoyed by the rest of society. In an era of cutback government, severely disabled persons are not singled out. Cutbacks, when implemented, are usually considered in the framework of how all persons in society have been affected by the current economic downturn. Such thinking does not exist in the United States where there have always been persistent doubts about persons who depend on the public's largess for their well-being.

However, the high level of support in the Netherlands is also accompanied by a subtle but unmistakable paternalism that compromises self-direction and lowers the expectations made of persons with disabilities. More is often expected of a disabled person in the United States but often without the resources and without the benefit of a fully accessible environment.

Trying to obtain the best of both worlds is a difficult task. By considering the IL status of disabled persons in the Netherlands, this monograph has sought to obtain a better understanding of those factors that can also enhance opportunities for persons with disabilities in the United States.

SOURCES

Andeweg, R.G., van der Tak, Th., and Dittrich, K.
1980   "Government Formation in the Netherlands." *The Economy and Politics of the Netherlands Since 1945*, R.T. Griffiths, ed. The Hague: Martinus Nijhoff, 223-249.

Brenton, M.
1982   "Changing Relationships in Dutch Social Services." *Journal of Social Policy*, 11 (January), 59-60.

Brand, W.
1980   "The Legacy of Empire." *The Economy and Politics of the Netherlands Since 1945*, R. T. Griffiths, ed. The Hague: Martinus Nijhoff, 251-275

Buijk, C. A.
1980   *Aangepast Wonen*. Amsterdam: Vrije Universiteit, Laboratium voor Toegepaste Psychologie.

Centraal Bureau voor de Statistiek
1983   *Statistisch Zakboek, 1983*. 's-Gravenhage: Staatsuitgeverij (October).

Centraal Planbureau
1982   *Macro Economische Verkenning, 1983*. 's-Gravenhage: Staatsuitgeverij (September).

Centrale Raad voor Gezinsverzorging
1983   "Inzake Gegevens Ontleend aan de Subsidieberekeningen van de Instellingen voor Gezinsverzorging over de 13e Administratieve Periode 1982." (Informatiebulletin nr. 14.) Utrecht: Stichting Centrale Raad voor Gezinsverzorging.

CRM (Ministerie van Cultuur, Recreatie, & Maatschappelijk Werk)
1980   "Social Policy Relating to the Disabled in the Netherlands." Rijswijk, the Netherlands: CRM.

Daalder, H.
1984   "On the Origins of the Consociational Democracy Model." *Acta Politica 19* (January) No. 1., 97-116.

---

1. *These references follow the convention used in most English speaking countries whereby authors' names are listed alphabetically according to the very first letter of the last name even when the last name starts with a lower case letter. The Dutch convention is to list authors alphabetically according to the first uppercase letter in the last name following a lowercase preposition (as in* van den Berg*).*

de Beus, J. and van den Doel, H.
1980   "Interest Groups in Dutch Domestic Politics." *The Economy and Politics of the Netherlands Since 1945*, R. T. Griffiths, ed. The Hague: Martinus Nijhoff, 163-197.

DeJong, G.
1979   *The Movement for Independent Living: Origins, Ideology, and Implications for Disability Research.* East Lansing, Michigan: Michigan State University, University Center for International Rehabilitation.

de Kleijn—de Vrankrijker, M.W.
1976   *The Physically Handicapped in the Netherlands.* Voorburg, the Netherlands: Centraal Bureau voor de Statistiek.

de Wolff, P. and Driehuis, W.
1980   "A Description of Post War Economic Developments and Economic Policy in the Netherlands." *The Economy and Politics of the Netherlands Since 1945*, R. T. Griffiths, ed. The Hague: Martinus Nijhoff, 13-60.

Ellemers, J. E.
1984   "Pillarization as a Process of Modernization." *Acta Politica* 19 (January) No. 1, 129-144.

Emanuel, H., Halberstadt, V. and Petersen, C.
1980   "Cross National Disability Study: The Netherlands." Leiden, the Netherlands: University of Leiden, Center for Research in Public Economics.

Frijda, J.S.
1983   "Zelfredzaamheid," *Katernen Gezinsverzorging nr. 5.* Utrecht: Stichting Centrale Raad voor Gezinsverzorging, (March).

Gading Aktiviteiten Centrum
1983   "Programma 83." Leiderdorp, the Netherlands (mimeo).

Galjaard, H.
1981   *Het Leven van de Nederlander.* Utrecht: Projektontwikkeling Kluwer Algemene Boeken Utrecht.

GMD (Gemeenschappelijke Medische Dienst)
1981a *Jaarverslag 1980 (Algemeen Deel).* Amsterdam: Gemeenschappelijke Medische Dienst.
1981b *Jaarverslag 1980 (Statistisch Deel).* Amsterdam: Gemeenschappelijke Medische Dienst.
(no date) *GMD: Dienstverlening in de Praktijk.* Amsterdam: Gemeenschappelijke Medische Dienst.

Heijl, M., Hofberg, G., Hurtig, E., Jones, G., Paulsson, J., Schulz, S., Sundberg, S.

1983 *Housing for the Handicapped in Holland*. Goteborg, Sweden: Chalmers University of Technology, School of Architecture, Department of Housing Design, (October). Based on a Symposium held in Lunteren, the Netherlands, May 7-14.

Interministerial Steering Group on Disability Policy

1981 *Outline of the Present Situation with Regard to Rehabilitation Policy*. Based on two memoranda submitted to the (Tweede Kamer) Lower House of Parliament in 1977 and 1978 with updated material in the appendices. Leidschendam, the Netherlands: Ministry of Health and Environmental Protection.

Irwin, G.A.

1980 "Patterns of Voting Behaviour in the Netherlands." *The Economy and Politics of the Netherlands Since 1945*, R.T. Griffiths, ed. The Hague: Martinus Nijhoff, 199-222.

Jordan, A.G. and Richardson, J.J.

1983 "Policy Communities: The British and European Style." *Policy Studies Journal* 11 (June 1983) No. 4, 603-615.

Klein, P.W.

1980 "The Foundations of Dutch Prosperity." *The Economy and Politics of the Netherlands Since 1945*, R.T. Griffiths, ed. The Hague: Martinus Nijhoff.

Klein, T., and Meeus, J.

1984 "Heeft Fokus de Gehandicapten Totaal Geclaimd?" *de Volkskrant* (February 25), 9.

Landelijk Aktiekomite, Eigen Bijdrage, AWBZ

1983 "De (A)sociale Gevolgen Verhoging Eigen Bijdrage, AWBZ." Zandvoort, the Netherlands, (mimeo).

Lijphart, A.

1984 "Time Politics of Accommodation: Reflections—Fifteen Years Later." *Acta Politica* 19 (January) No. 1, 9-18.

Lubbers, R.F.M. and Lemckert, C.

1980 "The Influence of Natural Gas on the Dutch Economy." *The Economy and Politics of the Netherlands Since 1945*, R.T. Griffiths, ed. The Hague: Martinus Nijhoff, 87-113.

Muus, Ph. J., Penninx, R., J.J.M. van Amersfoort, F. Bovenkerk, & W. Verschoor

1983 *Retourmigratie van Mediterranen, Surinanersen en Antillianen uit Nederland*. Den Haag: Ministerie van Sociale Zaken en Werkgelegenheid (December).

Nationale Kruisvereniging

1983 *Kruiswerk 81*. Bunnik, the Netherlands: Nationale Kruisvereniging.

Nederlandse Federatie van Voorzieningscentra voor Lichamelijk Gehandicapten
   1982   *Documentatie*. Utrecht: Nederlandse Federatie van Voorzienings-
          centra voor Lichamelijk Gehandicapten, (June).
OECD (Organization for Economic Co-operation & Development)
   1983   *OECD Economic Surveys: The Netherlands*. Paris: OECD
          (January)
Schraven, B.
   1984   "Problem bij de Arbeidsongeschijkheidsschatting van
          Marokkanen—een Verkenning." Zoetermeer, the Netherlands: So-
          ciale Verzekeringsraad (mimeo).
Stichting Voorzieningen Gehandicapten Noordelijk Zuid-Holland en Corne-
lius Musius Stichting
   1982   *Jaarverslag 1981*. Leiden, the Netherlands: Stichting Voor-
          zieningen Gehandicapten Noordelijk Zuid-Holland en Cornelius
          Musius Stichting.
SZW (Ministerie van Sociale Zaken en Werkgelegenheid)
   1982   *Social Security in the Netherlands*. Den Haag: Ministry of Social
          Affairs & Employment.
   1984   "Social Security in the Netherlands: A Short Survey as per 1 Janu-
          ary 1984." *INFO*.
van den Berg, J. and Molleman, H.
   1975   *Crisis in de Nederlandse Politiek*. Alphen aan den Rhijn, the
          Netherlands: Samson Uitgeverij.
van Overeem, E.
   1984   "Terug naar de Inrichting?" *Elseviers Magazine* (March 10), 18-20.
van Schendelen, M.P.C.M.
   1984   "The Views of Arend Lijphart and Collected Criticisms." *Acta
          Politica* 19 (January) No. 1, 19-55.
Vereniging van Raden van Arbeid
   1984   *De Kleine Gids voor de Nederlandse Sociale Zekerheid*, 1983.
          Amsterdam: Vereniging van Raden van Arbeid.
VRO & SZ (Ministries van Volkshuisvesting & Ruimtelijke Ordening en
Sociale Zaken)
   1981   "Zelfstandig Wonen Lichamelijk Gehandicapten (het Clus-
          terwonen)," [Clusternota]. *Nederlandse Staatscourant*, (June 2)
          Nr. 102, 4-7.
WVC (Ministerie van Welzijn, Volksgezondheid en Cultuur)
   1983   *Mag Ik Binne Komen? Functiemodel Gezinsvervangende
          Tehuizen voor Lichamelijk Gehandicapten*. Den Haag: Distribu-
          tiecentrum Overheids Publicaties, (March).

APPENDIX

PERSONS & ORGANIZATIONS INTERVIEWED[1]

J. Beijers
Project Stockhorst
Enschede

J. Brouwer
Sociale Verzekeringsraad
Zoetermeer

G. J. Clay
Ministerie van Welzin,
  Volksgezondheid, & Cultuur
Rijswijk

S. Crost
Het Dorp
Arnhem

K. de Bock
Nationale Kruisvereniging
Bunnik

F.G. de Graaf
Gemeenschappelijke
  Medische Dienst
Amsterdam

H. de Man
Provinciale Kruisvereniging
  Noord-Holland
Haarlem

M. W. de Kleijn-de Vrankrijker
Ministerie van Welzin,
  Volksgezondheid, & Cultuur
Leidschendam

A. den Broeder
Ministerie van Welzin,
  Volksgezondheid, & Cultuur
Rijswijk

C.W. de Ruijter
Lucas-Stichting voor Revaladatie
Hoensbroek

J. Drente
Nieuw Unicum
Zandvoort

T. Fenis
Nationaal Organ Gehandicaptenbeleid
Utrecht

J.S. Frijda
Centraal Raad voor Gezinverzorging
Utrecht

J. Hendricks
Utrecht

M. Herwyer
Sociale Verzekeringsraad
Zoetermeer

G. Heykamp
Stichting Fokus
Ten Boer

G. Hunfeld
Gemeenschappelijke
  Medische Dienst
Amsterdam

G. Hylkema
Kruisvereningen in de IJmond
IJmuiden

D. Jansen
Ministerie van Volkshuisvesting, Ruimtelijke
  Ordening & Mileuhygiene
Zoetermeer

H. Jansen
Gading Aktiviteiten Centrum
Leiderdorp

D.A. Jonker
Ministerie van Welzin,
  Volsezondheid, & Cultuur
Rijswijk

N. Kanis
Project 20
Gronigen

J.P. Mackenbach
Ministerie van Welzin,
  Volksgezondheid, & Cultuur
Rijswijk

L. Markenstein
Nationale Kruisvernigen
Bunnik

L. Oostrik
Project Stockhorst
Enschede

C. Pels-Rijckln
Vereningen van Nederlandse
  Gemeenten
Den Haag

K. Pons
Lucas-Stichting voor Revaladatie
Hoensbroek

N. Pronk
Gading Aktiviteiten Centrum
Leiderdorp

---

1. *This is a partial list. It does not include many discussants met along the way, especially consumers and ADL assistants. These individuals were essential to the development of this monograph and are acknowledged here.*

P. Pulles
Nationale Kruisverniging
Bunnik

M. Riemsma
Stichting STREVO
Hengelo

L.C. Sijperda-van der Ent
Project Tweesprong
Emmeloord

A.M. van Beek
Nederlandse Gehandicaptenraad
Utrecht

S. van Egmond
Netherlands Red Cross
Den Haag

T. van Emmerick
Stichting Voorzieningen Gehandicapten
   Noordostelijk Zuid Holland
Leiden

J. van Engen
Woonvorm 's-Hertogenbosch
's-Hertogenbosch

E. vander Horst
Stichting Fokus
Ten Boer

J.F. van Leer
Nationaal Orgaan Gehandicaptenbelied
Utrecht

H. Veneberg
Enschede

E. Venema
Algemene Instelling voor Gezinverzorging
Enschede

J. Visser
Nederlandse Federatie van
   Voorzieningscentra voor Lichamelijk
   Gehandicapten
Utrecht

E. Wiersma
Stichting Fokus
Ten Boer

COMMENTARIES ON WRF MONOGRAPH #27: INDEPENDENT LIVING AND DISABILITY POLICIES IN THE NETHERLANDS, by Gerben DeJong

- Michael Herweyer
- Carolyn L. Vash
- Adolf D. Ratzka

Commentary: A Dutch Perspective by Michael Herweyer

This monograph takes special note of the competition between the various residential and independent living models. The roots of that competition deserve additional commentary. I would like to focus my remarks accordingly. Although the presence of the Fokus program has added a new dimension to the competition, it will be my contention that the present competition reflects a much longer standing set of conflicts that have their origins in competing value systems and in differing views as to how society should collectively respond to the needs of its most disabled citizens. There are 2 enduring conflicts that I would like to explore in greater depth: (1) the conflict between *mantelzorg* (environmental care) and professionalism and (2) the conflict between professionalism and consumerism.

Conflict 1: *Mantelzorg* vs. Professionalism

Near the middle of his historical survey DeJong introduces the concept of "private initiative" (PI) and the presence of PI agencies that sprung up in a society "pillarized" primarily along religious and ideological lines. As noted in the monograph, each "pillar" spawned its own network of proliferating PI agencies. Moreover, each pillar was autonomous in exercising control over its respective PI organizations. This administrative and programmatic autonomy was originally in keeping with its funding base: PI agencies were supported by private funds voluntarily contributed by each pillar's membership in response to the recommendations of each pillar's leadership, namely, its priests, ministers, trade union leaders, or various "well-to-do" and "enlightened" lay leaders.

The rapid growth and specialization of PI agencies, however, underscored a growing conflict between 2 models or philosophies of care. This conflict emerged simultaneously within each pillar, but did not not become an open conflict because the conflict could be addressed within each pillar.

The conflicting models or philosophies of care can be observed in the transition when care-taking functions—traditionally performed by family, friends, neighbors and others within a given pillar—were transferred to highly professionalized and specialized PI organizations. This development undermined the traditional system of *mantelzorg*, ("environmental care") and created a growing preference for the emerging system of professional and residential care.

Mantelzorg was direct and personal but in many instances was intermittent and even simply nonexistent. *Mantelzorg* was often provided out of a sense of duty that was continuously stressed by the family and other pillar-based institutions such as the church, trade unions, and political parties. By contrast, professional care was impersonal and objective but had strong paternalistic features. These paternalistic features arose from 3 separate sources: First, PI organizations were intially supported by voluntary contributions made by their respective memberships. Second, the boards of PI organizations were usually comprised of clergy, political leaders, and "enlightened" citizens whose standing in a class-oriented society was inherently paternalistic. And third, there was the ever-present tendency of professionals to know what was best for the client.

Eventually, increasing professionalization and specialization became costly and simply beyond the fund raising capacity of the various pillars. As a result, the PI system turned to the emerging welfare state for financial support. In fact, the PI system became an integral part of the welfare state. However, this financial relief produced a new source of tension: Increasing public subsidies and decreasing dues-paying memberships tended to reduce the degree of administrative autonomy to which the PI system had become accustomed. As noted in section II of the monograph, it took years of deconfessionalization and depillarization before the time was ripe to merge functionally equivalent PI organizations and reach some economies of scale. Extensive legislation and regulation were required to reduce the administrative and programmatic autonomy originally experienced by the PI system.

Concurrent with this trend was another development worth noting. Clergy and lay leaders who had traditionally occupied the boards of PI organizations were replaced by a new elite comprised of professionally trained providers, university-based experts, "spokespersons" for client groups, and later, clients themselves.

Conflict 2: Professionalism vs. Consumerism

Dejong rightfully pays much attention to the ways in which residential care and independent living are presently financed. In this regard much has changed. However, even these changes serve to underscore the larger conflicts cited above. When the public sector took major responsibility for the funding of the care system nurtured by PI organizations, the most common form of funding was simple cost-sharing where government agreed to pay for a percentage of the total costs. Later, simple cost-sharing gave way to rate-based funding (as in the residential care system) and eventually to entitlement-based reimbursement for services by an organization's consumers (as in the Fokus system). Although these shifts in the nature of public funding may seem subtle and small, they represent a qualitative change in how disabled persons should be perceived and how their needs should be addressed—no longer as clients but as consumers with legal rights and entitlements which guarantee a disabled person's claim "to a piece of the action," to use an American expression.

Thus, the concept of rights and entitlements represent a major challenge to the still very paternalistic character and autonomy retained by many PI-based organizations such as those involved in the residential care system. DeJong very clearly illustrates this new antogonism between newly enfranchised consumers and firmly established professionals in the last part of Section II and all of Section IV. For example, in the case of Holland's systems of policy consultation, the departure of the Dutch Handicapped Council or GR (*Gehandicaptenraad*), a consumer-based organization, from the provider-dominated Dutch Rehabilitation Association represented a clear signal that the artificially maintained antagonism between confessionalized pillars couild not cover up the new basic antagonism between consumers and providers.

In Sections IV and V, DeJong explores 2 different models of independent living: (1) the Fokus model with its system of centralized ADL assistance and (2) the one-on-one model of attendant care. In the former, assistance is provided along the more equivalent lines of a landlord-tenant relationship. In the latter, assistance is provided along the lines of a hired-labor contract. Both models can be regarded as expressions of a larger societal trend toward demedicalization, deinstitutionalization, self-help, and legally secured rights—or simply, consumerism.

Consumerism and Cut-back Government

DeJong observes that Fokus has enjoyed considerable success up to the present. However, past success does not guarantee future success in an era of cut-back government. In a sense, the future of the residential care system is more secure, not because of its brick and mortar fortifications, but because it is surrounded by professional legitimacy in the form of more highly trained personnel within its own ranks or among those it can call upon when consultation becomes necessary. By contrast, ADL assistants within the Fokus system and *alpha helpsters* within the home help system are usually young, nonprofessional, low-paid, and more transient labor and thus also a more easy target for government cut-backs. Cut-back government may very well prefer *mantelzorg* (environmental care) to Fokus projects. Indications are that the Christian Democratic Appeal (CDA), the leading party in the present coalition government, is strongly inclined to return to the classic model of *mantelzorg*.

Finally, it should be noted that consumer-based organizations, such as the GR, are not as secure or as powerful as they sometimes seem. The GR, which serves as the main watch dog of consumer interests, is still not well established in the whole concert of corporatist politics to successfully thwart any potential threats to the emerging system of independent living in the Netherlands. DeJong notes, for example, at the end of Section II, that the GR is still not represented on the Social Security Council. Yet the Social Security Council represents an important consultative body with respect to many of the benefits vital to a person's ability to live independently.

Given present political and economic realities, DeJong's suggestion to incorporate features of the one-on-one model of attendant care offers a promising solution that could simultaneously cope with the constraints of cut-back government and meet the independent living aspirations of Dutch disabled citizens.

U.S. Commentary, by Carolyn Vash

I agreed to prepare this commentary before I read DeJong's monograph. Had I read it first, I might have suggested finding a peer reviewer who disagreed enough to generate some interesting controversy. My marginal notes consist mainly of exclamation points. My overall reaction is one of admiration, as much for the tone of the presentation—which reflects compassion, moderation, and humility—as for the thorough, careful treatment of the subject matter. Actually, I'm not sure whether the invitation to serve as "peer reviewer" was extended to me as "Rehab Expert" or "Disabled Person." Since I automatically relate everything I read to both roles, I didn't bother to ask. As it turns out, the former got few chances to be hyper-critical and the latter wasn't patronized once. So, in the absence of opportunity for inflamed polemic, I'll content myself with highlighting some of the reasons for my positive reaction, elaborating on a few points, and picking a nit or two.

DeJong tells his story well. It is logically organized; the background facts provide a solid foundation for constructing a clear elucidation of the specific IL models and related approaches. These, in turn, support his conclusions and selection of features worth considering here. I'd read about many of the Dutch phenomena described and frankly found them hard to understand. I guess the problem was in the writing because from DeJong's pen they seem simple and clear.

In all honesty, what I liked most was the fact that his "implications for the United States" matched those which occurred to me as I read almost exactly. I strongly agree that clustered housing and centralized attendant services are good ideas—and not just for *other* disabled people. I wouldn't mind considering a Fokus-type arrangement myself—especially as my husband and I grow older. There are no retirement homes in my geographic area which accommodate elderly couples wherein one spouse is self care independent and the other is not (even when the independent spouse can provide the care). Such couples are routinely broken up and sent to separate facilities, not within reasonable visiting distance, with the differing levels of care. I successfully beat down the barriers to become a severely disabled member of the labor force as a young, now middle-aged, adult. But guess what? The struggle isn't over. When I become righteously *old*, I will confront a new set of barriers—and I may not be in good fighting trim. Those of us who will belong to the first substantial "generation" of aging working-disabled people need to start planning ahead. The Fokus model sounds pretty good as a way to start.

I agree also that the "residential" model is *out*, and that brick and mortar investments of this type can lock you into yesterday's ideas for a long, long time. And the devaluation of attendant care providers in this country must be addressed. We entrust to them intimate, crucial services which disabled people require to survive—and then pay them less than a living wage.

This is not a self-esteem-building message for either the providers or the people with disabilities. It says all too clearly, "We'd really rather see the less fit get 'selected out' but we're not quite ready to admit that." In 1980 the Los Angeles County Commission on Disabilities studied the salaries and wages for nursing attendants in the County hospital system and those providing in-home supportive services. The Commission recommended a substantial increase. Although the *issue* was not ignored, as DeJong claimed, the recommendation was. Hopefully, the Commission will not give up. Experimentation with a Fokus-type model could address part of the problem.

Concerning his chapter on "The Larger Demographic, Economic, Political, and Social Context" DeJong states, somewhat apologetically, that "Some may find this discussion to be a digression." At last, a nit to pick. Surely this apologia is unnecessary—he errs in imagining such tunnel vision exists. In the past, I've criticised certain international rehabilitation efforts for paying insufficient attention to environmental differences between the countries which develop approaches which seem to "work" and countries which might import and adopt them. (By "environmental" I mean the variables he cites, plus technological level, and physical differences such as climate and terrain.)

DeJong conscientiously analyzes the data he gathered as might a political scientist, an economist, and an anthropologist as well as a rehabilitation researcher. His grounding in diverse fields seems stronger than many of us can claim. And he understands that whether a seedling takes root depends on whether it's transplanted into compatible soil. He figures out when the soil might not be compatible. If the idea still seems good and potentially transferable, he suggests ways of grafting it onto an American system which is already firmly rooted. Examples of this include using either the existing VR or SSDI/SSI system as a base for developing single-source funding for most in-kind benefits, and strengthening the National Council on the Handicapped (in specified ways) to give the disabled populace more reliable bargaining power. Whether or not these specific suggestions will prove to be feasible, I agree that something close to single-source funding must be instituted to halt the buck passing we experience as interminable searches for similar benefits. Also, an umbrella coalition of disability interests—wherein the differences among various segments of the disabled population are hashed out first and a united front moves on to the next level of bargaining—seems essential. Future analysis and experience will have to guide us with respect to the mechanism—whether it should be reconstituting the National Council, strengthening an American Coalition of Citizens with Disabilities or League of Disabled Voters, or something else.

Although all of these features of the Dutch system seem worthy of consideration here, the Fokus model is the most exciting idea (to me) in the monograph. It strikes me as a bonus that it was a Swedish importation to the Netherlands and that we can profit from another country's "false starts" in adapting it. DeJong gives credence to the fact that still further adaptation will be required in the American environment because of our strongly individualistic approach to almost everything. It's hardly surprising that we came up with a one-on-one attendant care system coupled with independent housing. It also figures that I would prefer to continue my ordinary residential style and decentralized way of obtaining attendant and housekeeping services as long as **a)** I can afford it and **b)** my needs are limited enough that it's easy to find capable providers. If/when one or both of these provisos changes, I'd certainly like to know that a non-institutional option is available.

SPECULATIONS ON THE FUTURE OF THE FOKUS SCHEME
Comments by Adolf D. Ratzka

The purpose of these comments is to contribute to DeJong's discussion of the Dutch Fokus model with some experiences from a consumer perspective with the present Swedish cluster housing model which constitutes a further development of the original Swedish Fokus concept. From such a viewpoint it may be interesting to speculate on the future of the Dutch Fokus system, in particular, on whether it will remain the main non-institutional housing alternative for severely disabled people. In Sweden the Fokus scheme has undergone some changes and recent developments there may be indicative of the direction which Fokus in Holland might take.

From the material presented in DeJong's monograph it would seem that the popularity of Fokus with Dutch social service planners and disabled consumers is due, at least in part, to the limited availability of noninstitutional alternatives relative to the number of persons needing extensive daily assistance with their personal care. A quick look at some simple statistics will illustrate this point. In the absence of more up-to-date and detailed survey data, DeJong observes that there are "several thousand persons between 18 and 65 years of age who require extensive daily assistance with their personal care." Estimates here in Sweden indicate the number of persons between 20 and 65, who need a Fokus-type arrangement, comprise 0.12 percent of the total population (Mansson, 1982). Applying this percentage to the total Dutch population results in a figure of aproximately 15,000 persons between 20 and 65 who need personal care assistance of the scope provided in a Fokus-type setting. If we now add up the estimated number of persons living in large residential centers (800), small residential centers (525), and Fokus apartments (200), we arrive at a total of some 1525 persons who live in semi-institutional and clustered housing settings. Yet, an unknown number of persons in need of extensive personal assistance are living outside of these options where, according to DeJong, they have to rely on unpaid help from parents, spouses, and friends. Such an arrangement often entails severe restrictions in lifestyle and cannot be considered a viable solution in the long run. Returning to our figures, we have approximately 13,500 persons (possibly more) living either in nursing homes or depending on their families for support while a total of only 200 persons live in Fokus units. This relationship suggests an enormous pent-up need for independent housing opportunities. Under these circumstances, there is no way of knowing how much of Fokus' popularity in Holland can be explained by its intrinsic qualities and how much is merely due to rathe absence of alternatives.

The overwhelming lack of independent housing alternatives and the relatively short Dutch experience with Fokus might also explain why so little has been done in the way of a critical evaluation of this model. In this respect the situation in Sweden is similar. There public officials and disability organizations alike promote cluster housing as *the* solution for persons requiring extensive personal assistance. As noted above, the number of persons aged 20-65 in need of this arrangement has been estimated at some 10,000 which, for comparison, is more than 2/3 of all Swedish wheelchair users in that age bracket. The estimate has been made by one of the most powerful Swedish disability organizations and has gone unchallenged.

In comparison to Holland, Sweden has had a longer and more extensive experience with cluster housing. Presently there are approximately 1000 apartments with access to 24-hour attendant service. The first 280 units completed before 1970 are the original Fokus units. Through the political efforts of the Swedish disability organizations and the Fokus Foundation Swedish local governments in 1973 were charged with the legal responsibility of providing that type of housing. Since that date all Fokus units are operated and financed by their respective municipalities. Up to now an additional 720 apartments have been built which differ somewhat from the original Fokus concept. Cluster housing is no longer referred to as Fokus but as "boendeservice" which might be translated as "housing with service." To the disability organizations pushing for more *boendeservice* apartments the term "Fokus" has negative connotations and they claim that there are significant differences. *Boendeservice* in contrast to Fokus apartments do not share common bathing, laundry, kitchen, and dining facilities. Also, the units consist of fewer apartments now ranging from 5 to 10 instead of 10 to 15. The basic principle, 24-hour access to staff from a nearby common staff room remains the same.

Fokus and *boendeservice* have been in existence in Sweden for some 15 years now, long enough to provide material for a discussion of some of the inherent limitations of this solution. Since in Sweden—in contrast to Holland—community based attendant services are more widespread and more oriented towards supporting disabled people living in the community, such a discussion is facilitated by the availability of other independent housing alternatives which can serve as points of reference. One of these limitations is the possibility that the attendant who is assisting a resident can be summoned to help another resident whose needs are considered more pressing. During morning hours the staff can seldom stay during the entire routine without interruptions, particularly, if some workers have called in sick and no substitutes have been found. Also, due to the high turnover—in some units up to 100 per cent—the resident can be faced any morning with a new staff member which has to be taught the routine. There might be so many staff members that the next time a certain person comes, he or she might have forgotten the resident's particular routine. As a consequence, it is often difficult to predict how long the morning routine will take which may be a contributing factor to why so few of the residents hold full-time jobs in the open labor market.

The staff is recruited by the social services district office without input from residents or present staff. Many residents experience discomfort and even humiliation when they have to rely on persons whom they could not choose for tasks intimately related to their body and personal space.

Another concern to many residents is that staff members are often forced to set priorities in how to allocate their limited time to the residents' competing needs. With time many residents have learned to assess the probabilities of receiving assistance for various tasks at a given time and to adjust their needs to the staff's schedule. Another response is to try to gain a competitive edge over fellow residents by developing a pleasing, non-offending attitude towards the staff.

There are some recent developments which point to possible changes in the *boendeservice* scheme and its prominent position among Swedish non-institutional housing alternatives. (Some observers might call both Fokus and *boendeservice* semi-institutional settings which suggests the need of defining what constitutes an institution in this context.) During the last few years several residents in some of Stockholm's older *boendeservice* units have successfully negotiated for their own personal attendants who are not otherwise connected to the unit and who come in the mornings to stay throughout the entire morning routine. During the rest of the day these residents rely on the central staff as before. Residents who managed to get these personal attendants—usually persons with extensive need of personal assistace—reportedly experience the change as a significant improvement in their quality of life. They report increased self-confidence gained from a feeling of being in charge and being able to plan their mornings.

As a result of a seminar on independent living in Stockholm in December 1983 with participants from the independent living movement in the US and the United Kingdom, Stockholm's independent living group (STIL) was formed with the purpose of increasing the number of housing and attendant service alternatives for consumers of personal assistance. While STIL does not deny the advantages of *boendeservice* over institutions or parental homes, its members argue that *boendeservice* as a single, general solution cannot satisfy different, individual needs. Severely disabled persons, according to STIL, despite their common need of personal assistance are individuals with different personalities, social and economic backgrounds who have the same right to find their own way of living as their non-disabled peers. The flexibility implied by this right, STIL members claim, depends on two requirements: not linking housing and services into one bundle and state or municipal attendant care allowances directly paid to consumers to enable them to hire, train and, if necessary, fire their own attendants.

STIL's initiative has met considerable interest and also resistance—not surprisingly from the established disability organizations who are strongly committed to the *boendeservice* model and apparently feel threatened by STIL. One of the most persistent arguments against STIL's proposed attendant care model is the contention that not many disabled persons have the ability to run their own attendant care. These doubts are most often advanced by social services professionals and by non-disabled functionaries of disability organizations. When pointing to the documented success of the independent living attendant model in the US, the reply is often that in Sweden there is a different social climate where local governments are strongly committed to supplying such services both financially and administratively. Swedish law in this area (socialtjänstlagen) counts the disabled among the "weak" groups in society together with children, the elderly, immigrants, etc. whose special protection local governments are charged with. As it is often put, "in Sweden we take care of each other." In this climate the independent living attendant model is seen as a necessity in the US to which disabled people in Sweden do not have to be exposed to.

While *boendeservice* has its rightful place among the present limited housing and attendant care alternatives in Sweden, these recent developments indicate that consumers there have begun to question the monopoly position this solution has had for so long. The hypothesis is here suggested that when the number of *boendeservice* apartments in a given community increases beyond a certain level relative to the number of persons in need of personal assistance, the only other alternative for many—a nursing home—ceases to serve as a reference point and other thinkable solutions are explored that promise more degrees of freedom. Perhaps it is no coincidence that STIL was founded in Stockholm which is the city with most *boendeservice* apartments per capita in Sweden—presently 120 apartments, more are planned—in a total population of some 600,000 inhabitants. It can be expected that *boendeservice* will lose its present prominent position and become one of several alternatives as soon as more flexible solutions as propagated by STIL are sanctioned and supported by local governments and the disability organizations.

REFERENCES

Mansson, K.C., *Housing with Day and Night Service for the Severely Disabled*, The Swedish Institute for the Handicapped, Stockholm, 1982.

Ratzka, A.D., "Community-Based Attendant Services in Sweden," in *Rehabilitation/WORLD*, Summer 1982.

WORLD REHABILITATION FUND, INC.
400 East 34th Street
New York, NY 10016

Howard A. Rusk, M.D.,
Chairman of the Board

Howard A. Rusk, Jr.
President
James F. Garrett, Ph.D.,
Executive Vice President,
and Principal Investigator

Diane E. Woods,
Project Director

Theresa Brown,
Project Secretary

Sylvia Wackstein,
Secretary-Treasurer, WRF

COOPERATING INTERNATIONAL ORGANIZATIONS
(U.S. Based)

University Centers for
International Rehabilitation
  William D. Frye, Ph.D.,
    Director, Michigan State
    University, Michigan

Rehabilitation International
U.S.A.
  Philip Puleio, Ph.D.,
  New York

Rehabilitation International
  Norman Acton, Secretary
  General, New York

Partners of the Americas
  Gregg Dixon, Director
  Washington, DC

INTERNATIONAL ADVISORY COUNCIL

Luis Vales Ancoma, M.D.
  Mexico
Diane de Castellane
  Paris, France
Professor Olle Hook, M.D.
  Goteborg, Sweden
Kurt-Alfons Jochheim, M.D.
  Federal Republic of
  Germany
Dr. Birgit Dyssegaard
  Denmark

Aulikki Kananoja
  Helsinki, Finland
Barbara Keller
  Zurich, Switzerland
Yoko Kojima, Ph.D.,
  Professor
  Tokyo, Japan
Douglas Limberick
  Australia
Armand Maron, Ph.D.
  Belgium

Sulejman Masovic
  Zagreb, Yùgoslavia
C.W. de Ruijter
  Hoensbroek, Netherlands
Jack Sarney
  Canada
Teesa Selli Serra
  Rome, Italy
George Wilson
  London, England

INTERNATIONAL EXCHANGE OF EXPERTS
AND INFORMATION IN REHABILITATION
PEER REVIEW UTILIZATION PANEL
(U.S. ADVISORY COUNCIL)

Sheila Akabas, Ph.D.
Director
  Industrial Social Welfare
  Center
  The Columbia University
  School of Social Work
Thomas P. Anderson, M.D.
  Department of Physical
  Medicine and
  Rehabilitation
  University of Minnesota

Donn Brolin, Ph.D.,
  Professor
  University of
  Missouri-Columbia
Richard E. Desmond, Ph.D.
  Chairman
  Department of Special
  Education &
  Rehabilitation

Ruth R. Green,
  Administrator
  N.Y. League for the
  Hard of Hearing
Gini Laurie
  Rehabilitation Gazette
Dr. Kenneth Mitchell
  Private Consultant
  to Industry

Dr. Mark Fuhrer
  Texas Institute for
  Rehabilitation
  and Research
Claude A. Myer, Director
  Division of Vocational
  Rehabiliation Services

Carolyn Vash, Ph.D.
  Planning Systems
  International, Inc.

SPECIAL CONSULTANTS TO PROJECT:

Leonard Diller, Ph.D.
  Institute of
  Rehabilitation Medicine
  NYU Medical Center

John Muthard, Ph.D.
  Rehabilitation
  Research Institute
  University of Florida

MONOGRAPHS IN THE SERIES´

Project Year 1978-80

#1 Readaptation After myocardial Infarction
Harold Sanne, M.D.
Goteborg, Sweden

#2 Hospital Based Community Support
Services for Recovering Chronic Schizophrenics:
The Experience at Lillhagen Hospital, Goteborg,
Sweden
Sven-Jonas Dencker, M.D.
Lillhagen Hospital
Sweden

#3 Vocational Training for Independent Living
Trevor R. Parmenter, B.A.
Macquarie University
Australia

#4 The Value of Independent Living: Looking at
Cost Effectiveness in the U.K. (Issues for
Discussion in the U.S.)
Jean Simkins
The Economist Intelligence Unit
London, England

#5 Attitudes and Disabled People: Issues for
Discussion
Vic Finkelstein, B.A.
The Open University
Great Britain

#6 Early Rehabilitation at the Work Place
Aila Jarvikoski
Rehabilitation Foundation
Helsinki

#7 The Role of Special Education in an Overall
Rehabilitation Program
Birgit Dyssegaard
Denmark

Project Year 1980-81

#8 Justice, Liberty, Compassion: Analysis of
and Implications for ''Humane'' Health Care and
Rehabilitation in the U.S. (Some Lessons from
Sweden)
Ruth Purtilo, Ph.D.
U.S.

#9 Rehabilitation Medicine: The State of the
Art
Alex Chantraine, M.D.
Switzerland

#10 Interchange of American and European
Concepts of Independent Living and Consumer
Involvement of and by Disabled People
Gini Laurie
Editor, Rehabilitation Gazette
and
Lex and Joyce Frieden
Houston, Texas

#11 The Prevention of Pressure Sores for
Persons with Spinal Cord Injuries
Philip C. Noble
Royal Perth Hospital
Australia

#12 Systems of Information in Disability and
Rehabilitation
Dr. Philip H.N. Wood
U.K.

#13 Verbotonal Method for Rehabilitation
People with Communication Problems
Dr. Carl Asp
University of Tennessee
and
Dr. Petar Gurbina
Yugoslavia

Project Year 1981-82

#14 Childhood Disability in the Family
Dr. Elizabeth Zucman
France

#15 A National Transport System for Severely
Disabled Persons—A Swedish Model
Birger Roos
Sweden

#16 The Clinical Attitude in Rehabilitation: A
Cross-Cultural View
Joseph Stubbins, Ph.D.
U.S.

#17 Information Systems on Technical Aids for
the Disabled
James F. Garrett, Ph.D., Editor
U.S. (WRF)

Project Year 1982-83

#18 International Approaches to Issues in
Pulmonary Disease
Irving Kass, M.D., Editor
U.S.

#19 Australian Approaches to Rehabilitation in
Neurotrauma and Spinal Cord Injury
James F. Garrett, Ph.D., Editor
U.S. (WRF)

#20 Work Site Adaptations for Workers with
Disabilities: A Handbook from Sweden
Gerd Elmfeldt, et al.
Sweden

#21 Rehabiliation in Australia: U.S.
Observation
Diane E. Woods, Editor
U.S. (WRF)

#23 Methods of Improving Verbal and Psychological Development in Children with Cerebral Palsy in the Soviet Union
L.A. Danilova
USSR

Project Year 1983-84

#24 Language Rehabiliation After Stroke: A Linguistic Model
Dr. Gunther Peuser
Federal Republic of Germany

#25 Societal Provision for the Long-Term Needs of the Mentally and Physically Disabled in Britain and in Sweden Relative to Decision-Making in Newborn Intensive Care Units
Ernle W.D. Young, Ph.D.
U.S.

#26 Community-Based Rehabiliation Services: The Experience of Bacolod, Philippines and the Asia/Pacific Region
Dr. Antonio O. Periquet
The Philippines

#27 Three Models of Independent Living in the Netherlands
Gerben DeJong, Ph.D.
U.S.

#28 The Future of Work and Disabled Persons
Paul Cornes
U.K.
and
Harlan Hahn, Ph.D.
U.S.

#29 Issues of Equality: European Perceptions of Employment Policy and Disabled Persons
Harlan Hahn, Ph.D.

The following monographs are still available (*or will be*) in limited supplies: #12, #14, #15, #16, #17, #18, #20, #21, #24-29.